RESET NOUR

As one of Australia's leading diet[...]
for her extensive knowledge of food, eating behaviour and weight control. Holding honours degrees in both Nutrition & Dietetics and Psychology, plus a Master's of Coaching Psychology, Susie specialises in weight control for women during perimenopause and fuelling for top executive performance. Susie is one half of Australia's number one nutrition podcast, *The Nutrition Couch*. Over her career, Susie has worked as a paediatric dietitian at The Children's Hospital at Westmead, as a sports dietitian with several elite sporting teams including the Parramatta Eels, St George Illawarra Dragons and Sydney University Sport, and was the resident dietitian with Channel 7's *Sunrise* for 12 years. As mum to twin boys, Gus and Harry, Susie is kept busy retrieving their rugby and soccer balls and building Lego houses.

Globally recognised dietitian and nutritionist **Leanne Ward** has over a decade of experience in the nutrition industry. With a background in clinical dietetics, she brings specialist expertise in the areas of fat loss for women, emotional and non-hungry eating, hormone health and digestive health. As The Fitness Dietitian, Leanne has over 700,000 followers online and runs two multi-national businesses, the Lean Gut Mind Method coaching program and the Leanne Ward Nutrition virtual clinic, to help people access experienced and accredited dietitians from anywhere in the world. As the other half of *The Nutrition Couch* and host of her own *Leanne Ward Nutrition* podcast, Leanne's shows boast a combined total of over 7 million downloads. She is also a busy mum to two young girls, Mia and Matilda, and loves her daily coffee habit, regular gym sessions and exploring new places when she can.

RESET

NOURISH

BURN

SUSIE BURRELL & LEANNE WARD

PENGUIN BOOKS

UK | USA | Canada | Ireland | Australia
India | New Zealand | South Africa | China

Penguin Books is part of the Penguin Random House group of companies
whose addresses can be found at global.penguinrandomhouse.com

Penguin
Random House
Australia

First published by Penguin Books in 2024

The information contained in this book is provided for general purposes only. It is not
intended for and should not be relied upon as medical advice. If you have underlying
health problems, or have any doubts about the advice obtained in this book, you
should contact a qualified medical, dietary or other appropriate professional.

Cover design by Smith & Gilmour © Penguin Random House Australia Pty Ltd
Recipe photography by Daniel Jokovich
Author photograph by David Ward
Typeset in 11.5/16.5 pt Calluna by Midland Typesetters, Australia

Printed and bound in Australia by Griffin Press, an accredited
ISO AS/NZS 14001 Environmental Management Systems printer

NATIONAL
LIBRARY
OF AUSTRALIA

A catalogue record for this
book is available from the
National Library of Australia

ISBN 978 1 76134 593 7

penguin.com.au

FSC
www.fsc.org

MIX
Paper | Supporting
responsible forestry
FSC® C018684

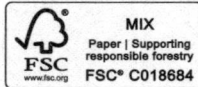

We at Penguin Random House Australia acknowledge that Aboriginal and Torres
Strait Islander peoples are the Traditional Custodians and the first storytellers of the
lands on which we live and work. We honour Aboriginal and Torres Strait Islander
peoples' continuous connection to Country, waters, skies and communities.
We celebrate Aboriginal and Torres Strait Islander stories, traditions and
living cultures; and we pay our respects to Elders past and present.

CONTENTS

INTRODUCTION

Hi – we are Susie Burrell and Leanne Ward, co-hosts of Australia's most successful nutrition podcast, *The Nutrition Couch*. We are so happy you've picked up *Reset, Nourish, Burn* – an inspiring and practical guide to help busy women become their best selves. As practising dietitians we see very clearly, through the wide range of clients we attend to on a daily basis, that nourishing our bodies is the key to optimal physical, emotional and psychological well-being. With this book, we are excited to share our knowledge and expertise to help you build your ideal nutrition platform, so you can become the very best version of yourself.

We are both qualified nutritionists and dietitians who not only offer practical dietetics, but also focus on the psychology of eating: the research that supports weight loss and the many reasons why, as women, we often self-sabotage our best intentions. There's a lot of good science out there, but as busy mums ourselves, we know what you *really* need is the latest science translated into easy-to-understand health messages you can put to practical use, straight away.

Over our years of industry practice, we've witnessed diet fads come and go, so we know what works and what doesn't. We are passionate about helping people find *sustainable* results – not quick fixes. The world is rife with uneducated and biased opinions, which is why we're committed to bringing you evidence-based advice on how to live your healthiest life, both through our top-rating podcast, *The Nutrition Couch*, and now, this book.

This is *not* another diet book. Rather, it is a plan designed to help you create a sustainable lifestyle platform that supports you in achieving your nutrition- and weight-related goals, built on 10 simple but powerful principles. Based on our clinical experience, we are confident these practices will radically change your health in the short term and long term – *without* you needing to adopt a restrictive 'diet'. As each principle can easily be incorporated into your everyday practice, they will eventually become habitual and part of your well-balanced lifestyle for years to come.

As the title *Reset, Nourish, Burn* suggests, this book is divided into 3 parts: 1) the importance of psychology in achieving your health goals and how you can *reset* your mindset around food for success, 2) how to *nourish* your body in ways that support your wellbeing, energy and weight management, and 3) what you can do to achieve fat *burning* when that is your goal. To set yourself up for optimal long-term success we suggest following the plan in consecutive order, or if you have specific intentions in mind, you can jump straight into the relevant section of the book.

If you have picked up this book with the goal of losing weight, you may find it strange that we have left the fat-loss or 'burn' section until last. This is not by chance. In our experience, weight loss can and should be quite easy once you've adopted the right mindset, adjusted your habits and behaviours to match your goals, and have become consistent with nourishing your body. The problem is, the average person doesn't do these things. Without this strong base, people may find weight loss harder to initiate or maintain. To truly create a sustainable healthy lifestyle, you first want to focus on upgrading your habits and behaviours, then on fuelling and nourishing your body, and finally if needed, dropping additional body fat.

Our advice is designed to help you navigate real life, so it's practical, useful and realistic. Step by step we are aiming to build your toolbox, to give you as many strategies as possible to help you remain on track with your dietary goals, no matter what the situation. These include some of our favourite tips from the podcast, roundups of key ideas and useful tactics, plus 25 delicious and easy-to-make recipes with weekly meal plans for both the Nourish and Burn phases.

As clinical dietitians who specialise in weight control and hormone regulation for women, we see the same issues crop up time and again across our client base, particularly among sets of women who share lifestyle behaviours. Applying our observations and our learnings, we have created several examples of typical scenarios experienced by our clients and aligned these with 4 'archetypes' to help illustrate common dietary and lifestyle challenges.

These case-study examples are designed to help show you how to counteract common behaviours that prevent progress. The interesting thing is that most of us are often unaware of when we enact such behaviours in our own lives. Showing you how these play out in everyday scenarios helps bring them alive and can shine a light on where you might be adopting them in your own life.

The four archetypes aligned to these examples and outlined below are not an exhaustive list, nor hard-and-fast definitions, but they are useful for illustrative purposes. However, in applying them to your individual situation, realistically you may find yourself identifying with several different behaviours across a few of the archetypes, or picking and choosing from the behaviours and strategies across several different case studies. Great! These case studies and archetypes are simply a learning tool. We hope that by seeing a behaviour in action, you'll pick up a few useful insights relevant to you.

1. The exhausted mum 🛒
    - Puts everyone else in the family first and is feeling burnt out as a result.
    - Often neglects her own needs and lets others sabotage her progress.
    - Finds herself with too little time to eat properly, so skips meals.
    - Tired, busy and exhausted, she often eats off the kids' plates.
    - She tends to reward herself with treats after the kids are in bed.
    - She feels too tired to do any extra, structured exercise.

2. The burnt-out corporate worker 💼
    - Pushing long hours – up early and working late – she is burnt out as a result.
    - Often finds herself busy working or in meetings, so skips meals or eats at her desk.
    - Lots of mindless, stressed-out and emotional eating.
    - Constant extra snacking due to catered morning teas and lunches, plus after-dinner grazing and treats.
    - Weekly celebrations with work colleagues featuring heavy meals and alcohol.
    - Long workdays, intruding on time to dedicate to exercise.

3. The empty nester 🏠
    - No longer needs to cook for the whole family, so makes 'simple' meals that aren't properly balanced.
    - Constant snacking and grazing throughout the day with less attention on regular meals.
    - Too little protein and too much carbohydrate in her diet.
    - An exercise regime that may benefit from including more high-intensity aerobic efforts.
    - Not enough strength training to support her metabolism.

4. The 'I eat healthy and exercise but get no results' 🏋 workhorse
   - Eats nutritionally balanced meals, but portions are often too large.
   - Loves making new recipes but doesn't understand how to tailor them to her individual requirements.
   - Gets hung up on 'superfoods' and supplements that aren't needed.
   - Enjoys eating out regularly but neglects to compensate her usual diet to accommodate the higher calorie load of meals out.
   - Sometimes over-exercises and only takes limited rest days, which can lead to the feeling of burnout or overwhelm.

In reading through the client scenarios we hope you might experience a lightbulb realisation around things you may be doing in your own life. Once you're aware of your behaviours, you'll be better able to implement the suggested changes to counteract them, and soon you'll be well on your way to shifting your lifestyle and to seeing significant results.

Imagine in 12 months' time, looking back on this very moment. It's a year from now and you're feeling so grateful you found this book. You've absorbed its information, applied it to your life and taken consistent action towards your goals. You can now see the changes in your body you had wanted for so long. You can feel your body brimming with energy. You have confidence that radiates from within.

Imagine it. How different would you feel if your hormones were better balanced and your digestive system was working optimally? How much would your training benefit if you were properly fuelled for your workouts? How much better would your lifestyle be, improved by your expanded knowledge around nutrition and wellness? How good would you feel?!

The exciting news is that you are so very close to being in that place. This book holds the steps to help you achieve the long-lasting results you've always wanted. Using science to guide your journey and learning sustainable, evidence-based strategies that fit into your life without hassle, you will finally turn your goals into reality. Let's begin!

THE 10 PRINCIPLES

RESET

1. Ditch the diet mindset
2. Commit to healthy you
3. Success is a system

NOURISH

4. Nourish for energy
5. Nourish for strength
6. Nourish for optimal health

BURN

7. Find your hunger
8. Time your meals
9. Volume-eat your veg
10. Follow our fat-loss formula

PART 1

RESET

FIRST,
LET'S RESET

Before we do anything – lift a finger, change our diet, implement exercise – we must first reset our mind. Getting in the right headspace for health and weight control is *essential* for success. Let's use this Reset phase as a time to pause, take stock and restructure our habits and routines to be aligned with the goals we have for ourselves.

Chances are, if you have picked up this book, you have an interest in your health. Perhaps you're starting from scratch with no real idea where to begin. Or maybe you already eat pretty well and consider yourself 'active' but still can't achieve the results you want. Either way, it's likely that 'in theory' you know basically what you should and should not be doing. But still, it's hard! That's the thing about modern life. While there is loads of information around and we have a decent idea of what we 'should' do, getting it right is not so easy.

It's not easy because life is busy. It's not easy because health and fitness cannot always be a priority. It's not easy because sometimes *all* the information is just *too much* information. It's not easy because if you are a woman, and in particular, a woman looking after several other humans, whether colleagues, a partner, child or teenager, or even a furry friend, you probably feel pretty spent and exhausted most of the time. Especially if you have looked after these other beings for many years.

Despite the challenges, the good news about making any positive lifestyle change – whether that's eating better, exercising more or losing weight – is that once you start, you will start to *feel* better. Each day you improve, you will feel more energised and more in control. Each step forward, you will feel more confident in yourself and your body. In time, this will lead you to feeling more powerful within yourself and across your life in general. Naturally, when you feel better, you are better equipped to deal with what life throws at you.

When we truly understand the underlying psychology behind *why* we self-sabotage, know why we struggle to break bad habits and create new ones, and start focusing on solutions rather than problems, then we can begin to make real change. This begins with resetting our knowledge base, approach and mindset around health, weight and nutrition. From there we can rebuild a nutrition platform that will sustain our health goals over the long term, a place where good eating and regular exercise and feeling energised seems to come more easily and naturally. An optimal way of living. An enjoyable way of being. Sounds good, right? It's achievable and it starts here.

SIGNS YOUR LIFESTYLE NEEDS A RESET

- You feel you've lost control of your food intake and/or exercise.
- You are gaining weight each year.
- You regularly feel tired or sluggish.
- You often eat when you're bored, sad, stressed or emotional.
- You rarely experience true hunger and no longer feel joy from eating.
- You feel guilty after eating.

- You feel all over the show and wonder if your hormones could be off balance.
- You have been diagnosed with a new medical condition.
- You have low self-confidence in your clothes.
- You feel 'stuck in a rut' with your eating and exercise.
- You're sick of dieting, counting calories or restricting what you eat.
- You rarely shop ahead or plan your meals.
- You regularly eat out or order takeaway.
- You have no structured exercise regime.
- Your exercise regime no longer gives you results, or you no longer enjoy it.
- You have entered a new phase of life and feel ready to make a change.

Reset – a powerful place to start

Reset is an initial phase designed to set you up with the right headspace to make and commit to positive lifestyle changes and, more importantly, show you how to stay in the right mindset to make these changes last. As we break down the psychology of eating, we'll shine a light on how past experience and early programming can profoundly impact our behaviours and the surprisingly strong influence of our environment on our daily food and exercise decisions, which ultimately determine our health.

Reset comprises 3 core principles, forming the first stage of our Reset, Nourish, Burn approach. Reframing your understanding of and relationship with food and exercise, this phase will help you establish a powerful nutrition platform upon which to build a long-lasting healthy lifestyle. Throughout Reset we cover each of the following principles in detail:

1. Ditch the diet mindset
2. Commit to healthy you
3. Success is a system

Not only useful for kickstarting a new regime, Reset may also be helpful to return to whenever your lifestyle starts to feel like it's getting off track and out of control. Through what you're about to learn, you'll gain simple but effective strategies to support you anytime you feel:

- You've fallen off the wagon.
- Your environment isn't supporting your goals.
- You're lacking motivation.
- You keep self-sabotaging.
- You have a negative mindset about your health.
- You find yourself blaming others for your own struggles.
- You have perfectionist tendencies towards your nutrition.
- Your success systems are failing you.
- You are stressed, tired or burnt out on a regular basis.

Whenever you start to feel like this, it's a good time to review and reset your priorities, goals and habits. This begins by fortifying your mindset to support your success. Through Reset, you'll learn how to *enjoy* the process of committing to your health long term. Once you gain this new understanding, you'll find it easier to move from anxiety towards acceptance, and ultimately, to reach and maintain your goals.

CHAPTER 1

DITCH THE DIET MINDSET

When it comes to diet and nutrition, the reality is that there are simply no quick fixes. While there are plenty of fad diets, juice fasts and regimes that promise you 'so many kilos lost in a few short weeks', ultimately, when a diet or product sounds too good to be true, it usually is. Typically, after adhering rigidly to a new (often unrealistic) protocol you'll eventually go back to your regular lifestyle . . . and end up right back where you started – regaining all the weight you had lost (and often more) and still feeling none the wiser about how to eat well and maintain a healthy weight over the long term.

We see this time and again in our clinical practice. Clients turn up despondent and disheartened after having tried so hard to do 'everything right' yet getting nowhere. But it's not their fault. Each time someone begins another fad diet that promises the world, they are wasting precious time and energy. These 'miracle solutions' just don't work over the long haul.

There is nothing good that comes from the 'diet mindset'. Ultimately, the sooner we accept that eating well and moving our body is something we'll need to do on most days for the rest of our lives, the easier weight control becomes. Ignoring this fundamental principle is the primary reason most people regain weight once they come off a particular program: they have not yet understood and accepted that to maintain their results, they will have to eat and move in a certain way forever.

Our bodies are machines. They need constant care and attention to perform at their best. The older they get, the more tending they need, which means we must work harder to keep them running well. Over time, if we continually fuel our bodies with poor quality food, and too much of it, and don't keep them moving, it's no wonder things start to go wrong!

You know from observing those around you, it's the people who maintain key habits that positively support their health and wellbeing who are best able to maintain control of their weight over the course of their lives. These well-proven habits are based on a few key principles which underpin our approach. It is not a short-term diet program, but a long-term lifestyle.

This might sound like we've just handed you a life sentence – forever?! How dull! How restrictive! But actually, letting go of short-term 'diet thinking' and all the insidious beliefs that come with it is incredibly liberating. That's why this is the perfect place for us to start our reset.

Meet Louise: a chronic dieter

At 29, Louise's life as a corporate lawyer underpinned her relentless pursuit of perfection, especially when it came to her diet. She wanted a sculpted body and was eager to shed fat and build muscle, but her relationship with food was fraught with tension. Having previously done a bikini competition, she'd developed a poor relationship with food and a very all-or-nothing diet mindset. Her weekdays were a testament to discipline: meticulously portioned meals, each a careful assembly of one carb, one protein and one vegetable, all tracked in MyFitnessPal and driven by a deep-seated fear of fats and caloric load. To try to keep her food cravings in check, she constantly sipped on diet soft drinks.

Louise's rigid 'clean eating' left little room for enjoyment and led to a cycle of deprivation and over-indulgence. Come the weekend, having used up all her willpower, Louise would release her pent-up cravings by eating out for nearly every meal. Desserts and drinks were followed by feelings of physical and emotional discomfort, and her immune system bore the brunt of this chronic stress and poor nutrient intake. Louise was constantly rundown and often sick with colds and bugs.

Aware she was not feeling or performing at her best, Louise knew something had to shift. Having decided she wanted to escape the dieting mindset that had long dominated her life, she started seeing a dietitian. They agreed the first step towards change should be to stop using MyFitnessPal, as following it so religiously had distanced Louise from her body's natural hunger signals. Freed from its grip, she embarked on a journey of intuitive eating, learning to trust her body and to recognise portion sizes without external cues.

Mindful eating became Louise's new mantra as she learnt to savour treats in moderation, integrating them into her daily life rather than relegating them to weekend blowouts. She reintroduced fats into her meals and found that they reduced her cravings and left her feeling more satisfied. When the urge for something sweet emerged, she would partake mindfully, choosing to enjoy a small portion of what she genuinely wanted rather than reaching for a diet substitute. Louise replaced the critical voice in her head with positive self-talk, and she nurtured her gut health with an abundance of plants, fibre and prebiotics.

With this new approach, Louise learnt to see that every meal was a fresh start. She no longer felt she had to wait for a new week to eat well, and this helped soften her weekend excesses. The results were profound. Not only did Louise shed fat and grow stronger, she also improved her immune system and made it through 6 months without a single illness. Her cravings subsided, replaced by a newfound trust in her body's cues for hunger and fullness. Exercise transformed from a daily obligation into a source of joy. Louise had finally broken free from the chains of dieting, embracing a life where food was no longer an enemy but a source of nourishment and pleasure.

NOTES FROM THE NUTRITION COUCH
HOW TO SPOT A FAD DIET OR TREND

On social media, diets and new food trends are everywhere, so it can be hard to decipher what information is worth taking in and what to ignore. Here's what to keep in mind when assessing a new health plan.

1. Make sure the plan is created by a credentialled organisation or figure. As much as we'd like to trust every model or influencer with a diet plan, some may be blessed with genes that mean it is easier for them to stay slim. They may also be paid to endorse the diet or product.
2. Is the plan evidence-based? Does the person behind it have university-based qualifications in nutrition and diet? Is the plan backed up by academic studies?
3. There's no one-size-fits-all approach – everyone's body is different. Avoid plans that guarantee a weight-loss number in a set time frame or plans that prescribe the same foods or amounts for everyone.
4. If it sounds too good to be true, it probably is. Think of assessing a new diet like a potential investing scam – those massive returns (in this case weight loss) it is promising to deliver are probably too good to be true.
5. Is it a sustainable program? If the diet eliminates whole food groups or your favourite foods altogether it will be better for

your health long term to avoid it. Though short-term fixes are psychologically attractive, they are not realistic for our health.

If in doubt, it is always best to consult a qualified professional, such as an accredited dietitian or nutritionist.

18 July 2023[1]

Let's talk about . . . the weight-loss beliefs you hold

It's time to examine our beliefs around weight, food, nutrition, exercise and health. The way we think about things forms our belief system, a mental safety net we develop from childhood to help us make sense of life. We pick up and hold onto beliefs about the world and our place in it from all sorts of places and for any number of reasons – perhaps from observation, or from what what we experienced, or from what we were told by our family, society, school and the media. Some of these beliefs we are taught explicitly, but often they are formed subconsciously.

If they were embedded when we were young, they can be particularly powerful. As with any of our beliefs, our weight-loss beliefs may not be true, or even reasonable, but they can still hold us back from achieving our goals when we default to them. If losing weight has proven challenging for you in the past, it may be worth spending some time reflecting on what you 'believe' to be true around food, weight and exercise, and gently querying the validity of these beliefs. Are they reasonable? Could they be preventing you from achieving your goals long term?

Do you recognise any of the commonly held beliefs in the table below? If these ring true for you, perhaps it's time to replace them with a more objective view, grounded in facts. This is an effective practice we use with our clients: first, we help them identify the beliefs they hold, then help challenge them with more objective information.

COMMON BELIEFS	OBJECTIVE VIEWS
Weight loss is hard	Most things are hard when you first start out but with the right plan, preparation, knowledge and support, things will be easier. Progress builds momentum.
Weight loss should be hard	Mentally, we often position weight loss as harder than it should be. Building the right toolkit – knowing what to eat when and developing strategies to support you – makes it easier.
I can never lose weight	Almost all people can lose weight by using science-based, proven approaches to develop a personalised approach to weight loss that is enjoyable long term.
I will always be overweight	How you have been in the past is a result of the knowledge and support systems you had in place then. With a new approach and understanding, your future can look very different.
There is something wrong with my metabolism	Fewer people than you'd expect have medical issues with their metabolism. If you haven't seen any progress after following weight-loss guidelines, working with a professional will help you unearth any underlying medical causes.
Every time I lose weight, I put it back on again	Building a healthy mindset and lifestyle will help you manage your weight over the long term. It is entirely possible to lose weight in a healthy and sustainable way and keep it off for good.
If I eat less, I should lose weight straight away	Building a long-term healthy lifestyle approach to weight management may take a little longer, but it will also last much longer. Sustainable results are not instant.
Thin people can eat whatever they like	While we all have different body shapes, we can each affect our metabolism by what we eat and how we move. Learn what works best for your body to become the healthiest version of you.

So many people approach weight loss with trepidation and dread, which naturally makes it harder. Dietitians commonly hear from clients about having a 'last meal' – a final indulgent meal before beginning a new diet plan. This shows their perception that eating well and being in control of their weight will inevitably involve deprivation, hunger and eating none of the foods they like to eat.

Our approach is the opposite. We encourage our clients to eat the foods they love, in healthy ways and in healthy proportions for their bodies. Many indulgent favourites can be made healthier with a few simple tweaks but we also encourage you to enjoy the occasional treat as part of a sustainable long-term approach to weight loss. In addition, the more of these healthy changes you make, the better you'll start to feel, and this builds its own momentum. Soon you'll have more energy, feel better, look better and be more confident to continue with these healthy changes.

What is different when you commit to a lifestyle of balanced weight control is that you stop mindlessly overeating and over-indulging. You stop sabotaging yourself and eating poor quality food simply because it is available. You start to respect your body and nourish it with good quality food, even if it is occasionally a little higher in calories. You concentrate on what you *can* and *need* to eat to be at your best, rather than what you cannot – a simple but significant shift in mindset.

Where do your current beliefs come from?

The early experiences we had with food and diets can exert a powerful force over our relationship with food for our entire lives. In some cases, we are conscious of these influences – for example, perhaps we were told that we 'must' finish everything on our plates, so now we eat whatever we are served, regardless of hunger or appetite. Then, there are the other more insidious influences that can fuel disordered eating patterns for years of our lives, often without us even realising. For this reason, if weight issues have plagued you for much of your adult life, or if you remain unsure as to why your behaviour around some foods simply does not make sense, it may be time to reflect on how your early food experiences are impacting you now. Are they acting as a barrier preventing you reaching your health-related goals?

Reflect on your earliest food experience

A relatively simple technique that can reveal much about our early food programming is to take some time to recall and reflect on any standout food or diet-related memories from your childhood. Create some space and time to let your mind wander back to a certain age or period in your life – perhaps a key memory of a family celebration, a person, a house you lived in, or even a restaurant or meal out. When we place our focus on a food or meal aspect of a particular time, different memories will emerge, which may offer powerful insights into the messages we received as children about the role of food and eating in our lives.

They could be something like being told to stop eating so you 'don't put on weight'. Or your appearance being appraised by a family member. Or seeing a close relative obsessed with diets and restrictive eating. Or hearing constant comments about others' weight and appearance. Influences like these may have pro-grammed your subconscious to form a belief that to lose weight, you need to count calories and actively restrict your intake.

Why are such insights so powerful? When we understand the reason behind 'why' we may do things, it can be easier to accept and manage our responses. For example, in the case of eating everything on your plate, knowing this is what you have been automatically programmed to do helps you create mindfulness around eating what is served. In turn, this can help you consciously manage your appetite and become aware of not eating on autocue.

Or, in the case of following restrictive diets, knowing this was not *your* belief but rather what you were taught from a young age by those around you helps you see that today, as a self-directed adult, you can choose to let go of that belief.

Often when we find ourselves regularly engaging in dysfunctional eating behaviours – over-indulging when we want to lose weight, buying foods we know we will overeat, or mindlessly munching on foods we do not even enjoy that much – we will discover that the undermining belief or behaviour was set by our early childhood food experiences. In many cases, once you become more aware of these subconscious drivers, you will be in a much stronger position to acknowledge them, release them and finally move forward.

Perfectionism and failure – let's break the cycle

One of the most common food beliefs we see driving diet behaviour, particularly in women, is the idea that we must be 'perfect' with our diet to achieve maximal results. But starting each new day or week with a finely mapped-out plan or strict protocol around what we 'should' and 'shouldn't' eat can set us up for failure. If we don't perfectly meet our 'rules' this perpetuates a negative mindset. It is especially unhelpful when real life gets in the way of being able to follow such a restrictive plan.

Once the 'perfect plan' is violated, a feeling of failure sets in. This often results in giving yourself psychological permission to eat everything and anything. We tell ourselves, 'I've messed up, so might as well throw it all out the window and start again next week!' Then, after succumbing to over-indulgence and mindless eating, we decide to 'start fresh', only to inevitably 'fail' again, kickstarting the cycle to begin again, only this time often stricter because we 'failed' last time – and so it continues.

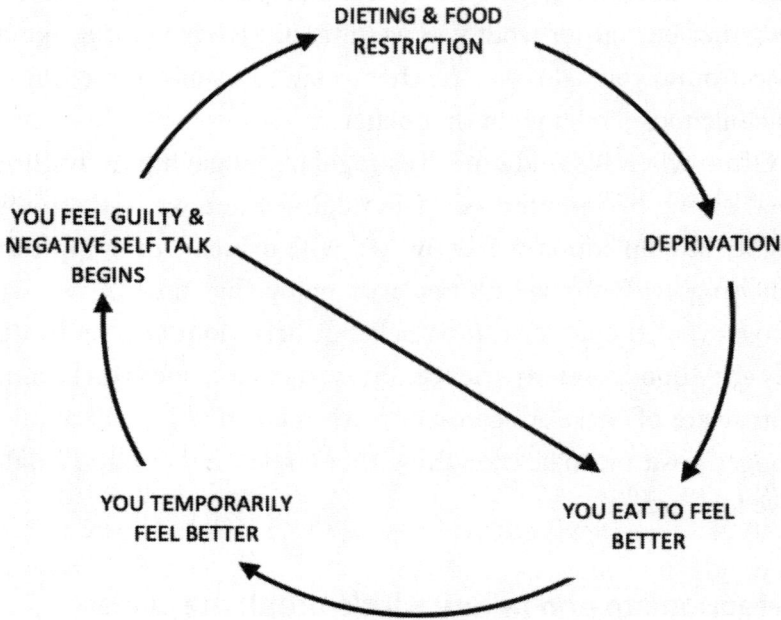

Whether we engage in this dietary psychological warfare with ourselves as a result of personal experience, self-punishment or early programmed behaviour really does not matter. Instead, what *does* matter is challenging the commonly held beliefs that your diet has to be 'perfect' for you to lose weight, and that the stricter you are with yourself, the better your weight-loss results will be. The bottom line is: this is simply not true.

To have a healthy and balanced lifestyle over the long term, the dieting cycle is the *first* thing you need to give up. It's clear it doesn't serve you – the more you restrict, the more you tend to 'fall off the wagon', beat yourself up mentally and maybe even add to your overall weight over time. The key to weight control is consistency, not perfection.

If you are a seasoned dieter from way back, it is time to get real and challenge these beliefs and put an end to the behaviours that drive this cognitive model of restriction, followed by overeating, over-indulging, self-flagellation and guilt, followed by restriction again. It is time to ditch the diet cycle for good. You have wasted enough time and energy on strict diets that do not work long term.

As you'll discover in later chapters, your true power lies in focusing on balanced meals, getting back in touch with your hunger and what you feel like eating, and listening to your body rather than trying to follow a strict set of rules that you have made for yourself or been given by someone else. Doesn't that sound like a much more enjoyable way to live? What's more, it works!

Why diets are so hard – the science

Through our practice we've seen that the women who successfully change their eating and exercise habits long term are those who set small and achievable goals, who are realistic about their goals and weight-loss expectations and who are intrinsically motivated. On the other hand, women who are less likely to be successful with weight loss tend to have unrealistic expectations and lower levels of motivation, and feel less satisfaction with their progress over time.

You might think that failing a diet makes you weak, but the truth is that, more often than not, it's the diet that failed you. Restrictive diets and rigid eating regimes are extremely difficult to maintain, and there are many reasons why they do not work long term, as the scientific literature suggests.[2]

Strict dieting is so hard because diets can:

- Cause mental fatigue.
- Make the brain more sensitive to stress.
- Increase cravings for treats or 'forbidden' foods.
- Lead to an all-or-nothing mindset.
- Be isolating and make socialising hard.
- Lead to an increase in over-indulgence when people fall off the wagon.
- Cause metabolic, hormonal and neurological changes.

- Cause disordered eating.
- Create feelings of guilt and shame.
- Lead to a regain of the weight lost (and even more, in many cases).

So instead of strict diets, we advocate a different approach: long-term change. As research supported by the Harvard Medical School shows, people who have lost weight and kept it off have usually made a permanent shift towards healthier eating habits.[3] Overhauling one's dietary patterns requires considerable mental and physical adaptations. As such, adopting a slow-and-steady approach to making lifestyle changes is more likely to deliver long-term results. Treating the process holistically – to include not only dietary adjustments, but also motivational support and lifestyle modifications – is generally shown to be effective, as our own and industry-wide case studies show.[4]

The best way to achieve this is to start by making small but consistent changes to your routine. Over time, these will become habits. No more 'falling off the wagon' and starting back at square one, over and over. It is time to get off the cycle and move freely into a much more balanced path ahead.

Creating your nutrition platform

We have now established that diets need to go, and with them, the cycle of restrictive eating and failure that leaves us feeling like we don't have control over our own weight and body. So, what's the alternative?

Adopting a sustainable mindset: being confident that your 'diet' is one you can happily maintain for a long period. The secret to this is designing a personal baseline diet that suits you. It should be built around your food likes and dislikes, fit into your lifestyle and be easy to maintain most of the time. It should regularly include foods you enjoy and allow room for occasional indulgent eating. However, it's important to be honest with yourself when it comes to treats.

Typically, we see too many treats and ultra-processed foods (UPFs) making their way into our clients' everyday eating patterns. These foods tend to have many added ingredients such as sugar, salt, fat and artificial colours or preservatives, as well as extracted substances like hydrogenated fats and additives like artificial colours and flavours or stabilisers. Examples of these foods are soft drinks, processed meat, fast food, biscuits, cakes, pastries, potato chips and other salty snacks. While big on flavour (and scientifically designed to be so, as well as ticking boxes for 'mouth-feel'), they offer little by way of good nutrition and are generally far less satisfying than wholefood options, leaving you hungry not long after eating them. Several studies have shown associations between UPFs and higher risks of cardiovascular disease, coronary heart disease, cerebrovascular disease and obesity.[5]

It's easy to discount the many treats we include in our diets. While in our minds we think of our regular meals and consider we are eating a balanced diet, we often forget to include the work morning tea with baked treats, the 3 pm chocolate or soft drink pick-me-up, the before-dinner potato chip grazing and the after-dinner wine or ice-cream. (And this doesn't even include the weekend treats . . .) It's not about always saying no to all these delicious foods, but instead adopting the mindset of balanced eating, where you aim to stick to your eating plan most of the time while allowing the occasional treat. This is enough to deliver results without stirring the emotions of guilt and failure and gives you the flexibility to respond to the realities of everyday life.

Balanced eating acknowledges that your diet doesn't need to be 'perfect' but aims to include as many nourishing foods as possible and focuses on eating well most of the time, as well as mindfully eating to nourish your soul. That's why we call fun foods 'soul foods'. There is not a lot of room for extras when eating for weight loss and weight control, especially once we take into account celebrations, eating out, and small treats like a little chocolate, wine or dessert. So when you do choose to indulge, do so intentionally and choose a 'soul food' – something that really makes your heart sing and your spirit soar, and make it count! Take a moment to really savour the flavour and enjoy the moment rather than, say, mindlessly munching on chips while watching TV or eating cake just because it's been put out. In practical terms, adopting a 'balanced eating' mindset is a manageable approach that delivers results.

Stay solutions focused

Keeping focused on your long-term objective is far more important than focusing on why you did or did not do something over the last 24 hours. If you do happen to get caught out, rather than dwelling on the negative, tune in to what you can do to make better decisions in the future and remember, you are in this for the long haul. Ruminating on the past will not get you anywhere. To get to where you want to go, turn your attention to what you need to do, step by step, one day at a time.

Being blinkered by restrictive diets often prevents us from seeing better solutions. Ditching the diet mindset frees you up to think more positively about your health, energy, lifestyle and personal goals. In the context of food and exercise, this means knowing what you need to do on a daily basis to keep on track. This may be as simple as taking food with you, or paying for a trainer, or as complex as pre-ordering special food when you travel.

Taking control of your diet and eating plan is about proactively planning, predicting and preparing so that you remain in control of your environment. For most of us, while high-calorie foods are readily available, 'convenience foods' are rarely the best choice and finding time to exercise can be a challenge. Replacing our 'diet mentality' with a sustainable healthy lifestyle will better support our long-term weight-management goals.

PLAN AHEAD TO STAY ON TRACK

- Meal-plan your week and batch-cook to get ahead.
- Double the recipe and freeze healthy meals for when you're short on time.
- Carry healthy snacks, like nut bars, in your bag for emergencies.
- Bring your own lunch to work (make extra dinner for leftovers).
- Before eating out, look up the menu and pre-plan your order.
- When travelling, locate the closest gym, running track or Pilates class to where you're staying.
- Have a back-up plan for your exercise session in case it's raining or cold.

CHAPTER 2

COMMIT TO HEALTHY YOU

The psychology of weight loss is complex, which is why so many people battle with their weight throughout their lives. On top of the mental load, there are genetics, hormones, habits, behaviours, lifestyle preferences, stressors and disorders to consider, making the idea of 'calories in vs. calories out' a tad simplistic. And while it's helpful to understand what issues may be impacting our weight – mental, medical or otherwise – the more important thing is to take action to manage it.

As we see in our clinical practice, there is one particular trait among those who do manage to lose weight and keep it off: they are committed to doing so. These clients present in a completely different headspace than those for whom weight control is fleeting. We find that for our successful clients, once the decision is made, there is simply no going back. They have committed to being the healthy version of themselves.

Typically, individuals who are successful in weight management refuse to accept failure. While they may fall off the rails occasionally or get frustrated when they have not lost as much weight as they would have liked, in general, once they've decided to lose weight, they will do whatever it takes. If it means not drinking any alcohol, they do it; if it means training at the gym every day, they do it. Because they *expect* to lose weight, their strong mindset helps them get there. And this same attitude helps them keep it off, too.

The reality is, there will always be food-based celebrations, treats at work, holidays and parties. There will always be reasons to skip the gym and eat more than you should – that's life! If we are to take control, we must also accept that it's up to us to manage our eating behaviour, and not just when we have a big hole in our social calendar (which, as we know, rarely happens!). It's the kind of self-management that can be learnt, and once you understand and accept it, managing your weight in day-to-day life becomes much easier.

Rather than letting our weight and weight issues control us, we need to take control of them. We need to stop blaming other things or people and make the changes we need to make, now. Not next week, when you are organised, and not next month when the birthdays are over! Now is your moment – seize it!

Meet Sanna: recognising self-sabotage 🛒

Sanna, a 33-year-old mother, was determined to reclaim her health amid the chaos of parenting. With a toddler in tow and the lingering effects of post-pregnancy weight, she and her partner, Jonas, were united in their commitment to a healthier lifestyle to achieve their family's future dreams. Sanna's desire to alleviate her IBS symptoms, lose weight and prepare her body for another pregnancy was matched by Jonas's support and their shared aspiration to be role models for their child.

Their previous attempts at healthy living had been inconsistent. Generous portions, protein-dominant plates and the convenience of takeaway food were their downfall, as well as snacking during their evening routines. Their meals lacked variety, typically featuring a single vegetable, if any. The weight they both carried had been a constant throughout their lives, and the additional weight Sanna had gained during pregnancy stubbornly remained.

Despite these challenges, Sanna and Jonas decided it was time for a change and embarked on a transformative journey. They began by re-evaluating their meal prep to focus on creating enjoyable and varied dishes they looked forward to eating. They introduced an array of colourful vegetables and healthy fats to their meals and reduced their protein intake to more reasonable levels. They deleted Uber Eats from their phones, removing the temptation to deviate from their plan.

The turning point came when the couple addressed their patterns of self-sabotage head-on. They had an honest conversation about the need to support each other's goals, especially in the evenings when the lure of mindless snacking was strongest. They made a pact to purchase only mini-sized portions of their favourite treats, so they'd be less likely to over-indulge.

Mindful eating became a cherished part of their meal routine, allowing them to savour their food and connect with each other once their toddler was asleep. Jonas also sought the guidance of a dietitian, embarking on his own path to better health, which in turn supported Sanna's efforts. They found new joy in shared activities, like weekend walks with their toddler, which doubled as family bonding and exercise.

To bolster their commitment, they established a regular 'gym date night', leaning on the support of nearby grandparents to watch over their sleeping toddler. This weekly ritual, along with sticky notes of their goals scattered throughout their home as visual reminders, kept them accountable and focused.

The results of their dedication were remarkable. Within 6 months, Sanna had lost 14.5 kilograms, and her waistline had decreased to under 90 centimetres. Their food expenses decreased as they were ordering far less takeaway, and exercise became an integral part of their lives. They discovered the power of mindful eating, which helped curb their overeating. Sanna's IBS symptoms improved dramatically, a testament to their healthier eating habits and better portion control.

Together, the couple broke free from the cycle of yo-yo dieting and embraced a sustainable approach to health and wellness. They had forged a new path, not just for themselves, but for their family, and their commitment had delivered them the balanced and healthy lifestyle they had been longing for.

Motivation

Many of our clients come to us 'looking for motivation', but this term has several layers of meaning. At a basic level, motivation is the force that drives us to do something – in the case of getting fit or losing weight, motivation drives the behaviours that will help to achieve this goal. This drive helps set us on a path to a sustainable healthy lifestyle and commit to long-term change. But for this change to last, we need to harness the right kind of motivation. There are four types of motivation, and one in particular – identified motivation – is the one we want to ignite.

TYPES OF MOTIVATION

Extrinsic – I do it because I *have to* do it.

Intrinsic – I do it because I *love* it.

Introjected – I do it because I think I *should* do it otherwise 'this may happen'.

Identified – I do it because I *want* to do it.

Extrinsic motivation is doing something because you've been told you *have to*, for example, reaching a target weight in order to catch a flight or get life insurance – you basically would not do it unless you had to. Understandably, this type of motivation is rarely sustained. It's unlikely you would be reading this book if you were extrinsically motivated to lose weight.

Intrinsic motivation is powered by internal desire – for the *love* of it. In an ideal world, most of us would have the intrinsic motivation to commit to the lifestyle factors that help us to control our weight, such as eating well most of the time and exercising regularly without thinking about it. But this type of motivation is relatively rare – most people do not love eating vegetables over chocolate, or love the treadmill so much they would rather get on that than sit on the couch and watch TV. Yet, there are some for whom this is true. Whether they were 'born' that way or have developed this love over time, these behaviours have become so much a part of who they are that doing them makes them feel good and they love it! While becoming intrinsically motivated may be the end goal, to get there, we usually need to engage identified motivation.

Introjected motivation is more common in the weight-loss area. In this case, you know you *should* do it, but are only really doing it for fear of something negative happening if you do not. For example, thinking you 'must' lose weight to avoid getting diabetes or to appease a partner or a family member. Again, this drive is not coming from within, so although it may be maintained for a while, it's difficult to sustain over time.

Identified motivation drives our behaviour from a place of *wanting* to do something because we know the benefits outweigh the negatives. We may want to eat a certain way and exercise to lose or control our weight and that strong desire comes from within – for example, getting up every day without fail to exercise as you know this supports your goals for your weight or your mood.

Often we can be driven by a combination of introjected and identified motivations; that is, you feel you *should*, to avoid negative consequences and you also *want* to, because you understand the benefits. Both these motivations are strengthened by the drive to give your lifestyle habits greater personal meaning. As stated in Gardner's paper on habit formation for health: developing habits you enjoy and feel good about implementing is the secret to keeping you motivated in the long term.[6]

When our motivation is not self-directed, it can be difficult to maintain. In the case of diet and exercise behaviours, this is one of the key reasons we fail long term: our goals are not being driven by our own energy and personal motivations, but instead by external factors. Understanding the factors that underpin your drive to do certain things or behave in certain ways – for example making healthy choices over unhealthy ones – can be helpful as you strive to reclaim your own motivation, rather than find it in external sources.

Individuals will be motivated by different things at different times. Some people are more inclined to eat well and exercise every single day, intrinsically motivated to do so as health and wellbeing is of high value to them. This may be something they were taught at a young age, are naturally interested in, or adopted after observing other fit and healthy individuals' success. Intrinsically motivated people rarely need support or guidance when it comes to health and fitness; rather, they are often on the lookout for ways to continue to improve and enhance their physical health.

If this is not you, and you find it tricky to locate and maintain your motivation around weight control, it's likely that you are still relying on external factors to spur you on. It may be worth taking some time to consider where your motivation currently sits, specifically in regards to health, fitness and nutrition. Once you've identified your current script, consider how you could reframe your health goals to give them greater personal meaning which will help them become more powerful. To identify the reasons why actively committing to a healthy lifestyle is important to you, you need to tap into your *why*.

Finding your why

The ability to link our diet and lifestyle goals to something bigger in our lives, a deeper why, is paramount in creating goals with strong meaning that can support and drive behaviour long term – just as Sanna and Jonas did in the example above, with their focus on their family's future. Identifying your personal drivers will help shift your motivation from introjected to identified, which is more likely to see it become a natural part of your life rather than requiring ongoing effort to maintain. Some common drivers that support identified motivation are wanting to live a long and healthy life, to be physically able to care for grandchildren, or to be physically fit enough to travel and explore as you get older. Everyone is different, but an easy way to help identify this type of motivation is to lean towards the things you find energising in life.

If you routinely struggle with motivation, make some time to consider why reaching your goal weight is important to you. To power up your motivation, spend some time reflecting on how you will feel once you've achieved your goals. Thinking about your optimal future in the present tense will help inspire your imagination and allow you to tap into how you will feel in that moment.

IMAGINING FUTURE YOU

- What benefits are you experiencing now you have managed to lose weight and keep it off?
- How are you feeling now that your body is looking, feeling and performing better?
- What is different in your life now you are comfortably managing your health and weight?
- What sorts of exercise are you happily doing every day?
- What sorts of foods are you enjoying eating and including in your daily eating plan?
- What barriers did you identify were holding you back and how did you overcome them?

Driven by values

Let's imagine that you frequently think or say that keeping fit and healthy is important to you, yet routinely find yourself failing to achieve the basics of eating well and exercising. Now, think about other things you do on a day-to-day basis and take a moment to consider why you do them – what value do they hold for you? For example, you may prioritise buying your morning coffee as you value the pleasure and energy hit it gives. Or you may take the time to message back and forth on WhatsApp because staying connected with friends and family matters. Or you may be able to find the time and energy to get your nails or eyebrows done regularly, as looking a certain way is important to you.

Your regular schedule can be a good indication of what is genuinely important to you, rather than what you *think* is important. What are those non-negotiables in your life, and what deeper value lies behind them?

On the flipside, recognising certain routine behaviours that may be less beneficial and understanding their perceived value to you can help you transition to healthier substitutions. Let's say, for example, you commonly have a glass of wine while making dinner, a habit you'd like to change. What you feel you gain from this may be: a quick way to unwind, the transition from 'work' to 'me-time', a palate cleanser, a thirst quencher or a way to bond with your partner. There are many alcohol-free drinks that could be an excellent substitute for this. Or if you want to break the connection altogether, finding direct replacements for each of the value points can help create new habits. For instance: unwind with a quick shower, transition to me-time by calling a friend, cleanse your palate by crunching on cucumbers, quench your thirst with a glass of sparkling water, and take a walk around the block to spend time with your partner.

How motivation becomes momentum

It is not uncommon for us to start working with a new client who reports they have 'no motivation'. By some miracle, they arrive with the expectation that simply by committing to a new program and paying for it, they will 'find' their motivation. Initially this may work. Investing time or money (or both) into a program can help kickstart action, but unfortunately this type of motivation tends to be short-lived.

Another mistake is waiting to 'become' motivated before we start something. In reality, the opposite is true. Daily habits create momentum over time, which in turn feeds motivation. This means that motivation comes from action, not the other way around. Most of us must keep mindful and focused to drive motivation. Consistently living a healthy lifestyle means habitually reverting to daily behaviours that are linked to our long-term goals.

Harnessing self-awareness

Once you've understood the deeper reason that's powering your journey to a healthy weight, it's time to take an honest look at your current food and exercise patterns to identify which areas require more focus. Self-awareness is the first step in identifying habits – both conscious and unconscious – that may be undermining your lifestyle goals. This may be especially relevant if you think you are already doing the 'right' thing and eating well but not getting the results you want to see. To get to the bottom of what's going on, ask yourself some deeper questions:

- Do I eat more than I need?
- Am I aware of hunger, or do I eat on autocue?
- Do I move as much as I think I do?
- When I am in the presence of food, do I mindlessly munch?
- Do the people around me negatively impact my food and exercise choices?
- What needs to change in my daily routine to support the health-related goals I have for myself?

Generally speaking, most of us have some idea of what our own barriers to success are, we are just not being honest with ourselves. Sometimes this is due to the associations we have made between healthy eating habits and feelings of guilt and shame, especially for those who have had a long history of dieting and not reaching their goals. In some cases, simply becoming aware of this inner script may help you highlight some of the changes you need to make, or you may need the help of a professional to assess your lifestyle and offer independent feedback on why you are not moving closer to your goals.

Don't be afraid to really question your past feelings, attitudes and behaviours towards food and exercise. Remember, in this new practice we have ditched the toxic diet-culture approach and are focused on building a loving, nurturing, supportive and healthy relationship with our bodies. Being honest with ourselves about our past, then giving ourselves permission to leave it in the past can be a helpful strategy for moving forward. It's time to disconnect your past behaviours from future you.

Self-monitoring

The easiest way to gain insight into your own behaviours is to self-monitor, which is one of the reasons dietitians may ask their clients to record their food intake. It is not to give feedback the way a teacher would on a child's homework, but rather to help gain insight into why, when and how an individual may eat and move each day, as when we are aware of our behaviours it is much easier to make changes. Self-monitoring has generally proven to be a critical component of sustained weight loss.[7]

However, when implementing self-monitoring, it is important to remain mindful of your primary objective. The foremost goal is to have a healthy relationship with your body, with food and with exercise. While self-monitoring tools can be useful, they are not suitable for everyone.[8] In some cases, self-monitoring can become excessive and it's important to avoid hyper-vigilance. If you notice that such monitoring is beginning to foster an unhealthy relationship with food and exercise, then it's time to dial it back.

Where self-monitoring can be most helpful is during the initial learning phase of implementing new approaches to weight loss. With regards to food intake, it may reveal that you are eating too much, or too little. Or, in the case of fitness , the realisation that despite 'moving' you are not getting enough exercise. Self-monitoring generates tangible data we can use to adjust our behaviours to become more in line with our goals and it's been shown to support the self-regulatory cycle of positive behaviour change. Specifically, when the goal is weight loss, self-monitoring of both diet and exercise behaviours is known to support better weight-loss outcomes.[9]

Self-monitoring can be much more powerful than being monitored by others as it helps to create ownership and agency over change, and as such, supports your drive to change in order to achieve your goals. Self-monitoring can be as simple as writing down what you eat each day or tracking your steps on your phone, or there are plenty of more advanced options that you can also invest in to help monitor and facilitate your diet- and exercise-related goals. Once you have the data to suggest which diet and exercise behaviours need attention and adjustment, you are in a better position to actively self-manage your lifestyle behaviours to support your health-related goals.

SELF-MONITORING TOOLS

- Food measurements: diet diary, portion control, meal-planning.
- Body measurements: scales, tape measure, callipers.
- Body composition: BIA (bioelectrical impedance analysis), DEXA scans.
- Visual: progress photos, tracking improvements in skin, hair and gut symptoms.

- Lifestyle: fit of clothing, mood and energy monitoring.
- Movement tracking: pedometer, smart watch or device, e.g. Garmin watch.
- Fitness: progress records, e.g. weights (max/reps), 1 km run, plank hold.

The above-suggested monitoring tools can be helpful to measure progress, especially in the early phases of working towards an ideal, healthy weight. Once you have reached this, often the most useful tool thereafter is simply using your clothes and general fitness. Find a pair of non-stretch jeans that fit comfortably at your ideal weight and try them on once a month to keep them from getting too snug. And set yourself a simple monthly fitness measurement – such as how long it takes to complete a 1 km run loop – to help monitor and maintain your fitness levels.

NOTES FROM THE NUTRITION COUCH
WARNING SIGNS TO LOOK OUT FOR

While we all have the best intentions when embarking on a lifestyle change, sometimes warning signs for eating disorders can arise. Ignored, they could lead to orthorexia nervosa. You may have heard of bulimia and anorexia nervosa, but orthorexia is a disordered eating pattern that is characterised by an obsession with eating completely 'clean' or 'pure' foods to the point it takes over your life and is detrimental to your health. If you notice any of these signs in yourself, contact a psychologist, doctor or dietitian.

- Prioritising weight loss over other health indicators.
- Consuming only health content that promises you will lose a certain amount of weight in a certain amount of time.
- Obsessively counting calories and tracking your weight daily.

- Eliminating food groups.
- Your sleep, skin and digestive systems are suffering – this can look like being constantly tired or cold.
- Skipping social occasions that may involve eating food you haven't prepared yourself.
- Obsessiveness when it comes to ingredient lists and all-or-nothing thinking when it comes to food.

3 July 2022[10]

The myth of self-control

It is a common misconception that diet and exercise adherence is dependent on being able to exert self-control: not accepting the cake when it is offered, not eating the chocolate in the cupboard, and setting the alarm to get up at 5 am every day and exercise.

While studies of successful sustained weight management show that self-control is important, what's shown to be even more so is creating environments and systems to support success. The use of healthy eating routines underscores the importance of self-control as both an automatic and deliberative process that is central to everyday decision making.[11]

When we take a closer look at research on self-control, while some individuals may score highly in the trait of self-control for lifestyle behaviours, generally, they are no better at resisting temptation when it is put in front of them, but they are better at avoiding temptation in general.[12] Specifically, individuals who are able to act in a more self-controlled way make it easier for themselves to be self-controlled as they develop strategies to minimise temptation. For example, if one of their goals is to not eat chocolate, they avoid going down the chocolate aisle when they are shopping.

This insight tells us a lot about the requirement to have self-control or act in a self-controlled way. To be self-controlled when it comes to both diet and exercise, the secret is to make it easy for yourself. Don't keep the tempting foods at home. Make exercise a part of your day. If you don't want to drink, don't go to the pub. One of the real tricks to building positive lifestyle habits is to spend a considerable amount of time planning, more of which we'll cover in the next chapter.

Let's talk about . . . self-sabotage

It might be munching on the kids' lunchbox leftovers. Maybe it's eating an entire block of chocolate after a day of healthy eating. Or it may be buying treats you know you will be tempted by, even though you are trying to lose weight. These are all examples of self-sabotage: engaging in behaviours that are not aligned to your goal.

Why do we self-sabotage?

An occasional slip is not self-sabotage – that's called being human! But when you find yourself sabotaging your efforts regularly, then it's time to pay a little more attention.

Like all behaviours, there are many reasons why people self-sabotage. It may have developed out of habit, or as a learnt behaviour over time. It may be that we are scared to achieve our weight-loss goals. Or, more commonly, it may simply be because we create an environment around us in which it is easy to self-sabotage.

Whatever the reason, if you regularly self-sabotage it is time to take a good look at your environment and find ways to make it harder. Do you need to throw tempting treats away? Do you need to drive a different way home so you are not lured to pick up a coffee and a cake? Or do you need to change your routine so you no longer associate a certain time or scenario with eating things you shouldn't or perhaps don't even really want?

For some people whose experiences with self-sabotage are more extreme there may be grounds to seek out further psychological treatment. But in many cases, it is about getting honest with yourself and finding ways to make it harder to undermine your bigger goals. It's time to make a plan for those times you find yourself vulnerable to self-sabotaging and to establish support in your home and workplace to promote long-term success. If you haven't had a conversation with your loved ones around how they can support you to achieve your health goals, now could be a great time.

Use this template and the examples to help you to assess the anchors around your self-sabotage and work out ways to avoid or overcome them in the future.

TRIGGER (WHAT)	LOCATION (WHEN/ WHERE)	PEOPLE (WHO)	STORY (WHY)	ALTERNATIVE SOLUTION
Snacking after dinner	In front of the TV	Partner	I want to relax after dinner	Watch TV with a herbal tea instead, or go for a walk together after dinner.
Eating kids' treats	Kitchen, preparing food or cleaning up	Me	I deserve them after a long day	Don't buy them as the kids don't really need them, or put them into a box at the back of the cupboard out of sight.
Over-snacking on the weekend cheese platter	Friend's house/in company	Friends or family	Everyone else is eating lots, so why can't I?	Offer to help hostess clean, or carry the platter around to everyone, or hold a drink so hands are full and there's less temptation to eat.
Continue to input your own scenarios in the boxes below				

TRIGGER (WHAT)	LOCATION (WHEN/ WHERE)	PEOPLE (WHO)	STORY (WHY)	ALTERNATIVE SOLUTION

Tips for committing to fat loss

We've spent some time discussing the psychological variables that underpin motivation, self-regulation and long-term weight control – all useful skills and knowledge to have for self-directed behaviour change. But when you have the specific goal of fat loss and losing a significant amount of weight, there is a high level of focus and commitment required, at least initially, to facilitate results. Here are our 4 top tips for getting into this mindset.

1. Get excited about eating well and caring for your body
Positive emotions such as happiness, excitement, joy, hope or pleasure lend themselves to generating more positive emotions. And the more positive we feel, the more likely we are to move towards our goals. It is not by chance that individuals who struggle with their weight are more likely to suffer from low mood.[13]

Getting excited about the future helps us open up our thoughts to consider the positives associated with weight loss, to see opportunities and to focus on the good things associated with weight loss. Dwelling in positivity provides less room for disappointment, frustration, resentment or annoyance – emotions that can prevent us from moving forward. Positive energy helps propel us towards our goals. Getting energised with your diet and exercise may be as simple as scheduling activities with friends, planning and cooking some tasty new meals or planning a new wardrobe – anything that makes you feel good is a great place to start.

2. Get clear on what you want

So often our clients want to lose weight, yet they aren't specific about how much weight they want to lose, nor about how and when they are going to achieve this goal. As such, they never get there. Instead of setting loose goals, like losing that annoying 'extra 5 to 10 kilos', or wanting to lose a 'significant amount' of weight, get specific. Decide upon an exact amount you want to lose by a set date. Firmly state your goal and commit the time and energy to achieve it.

As well as being specific, it's important to set realistic goals. As a general rule of thumb, it takes:

- at least 4 to 6 weeks to lose 3 to 5 kilograms
- at least 12 weeks (3 months) to lose 6 to 10 kilograms
- at least 6 months, usually closer to 12 months, to lose 20 kilograms or more.

The greater the amount of weight you have to lose, the more quickly you will initially see changes on the scales. For example, if you have more than 20 to 30 kilograms to lose, you are more likely to see losses of 1 to 2 kilograms *each week* on the scales, whereas if you have 10 kilograms or less to lose, losses of 1 to 2 kilograms *a month* are much more likely. When there's less weight to lose overall, the body has to work a lot harder to mobilise fat stores, so progress is slower.

Once you have realistic weight-loss targets in mind, consistent fat loss over weeks and months is about consistency and learning the difference between eating healthy and eating for fat loss (which we'll cover later in this book).

3. Go hard from the outset

A typical script from a new weight-loss client looks a little like this. Together we develop a food plan that will result in weight loss. Clients who follow it to the letter lose at least 0.5 to 1 kilogram in the first week they try to lose weight (if not more). They then feel empowered to continue with their weight-loss attempts and go on to lose a further 0.5 to 1 kilogram per week until they reach their goal weight. These clients have avoided alcohol, eaten mostly home-cooked meals, included plenty of fresh vegetables as suggested, and are delighted with achieving the results they expected.

Then, there are clients who come back after the first week and announce that they 'have been bad'. They still went out drinking on Saturday night, had a double scoop of ice-cream with the kids afterwards, and ate 3 chocolate biscuits after dinner most nights instead of just one. As a result, they have not lost weight. In fact, many have even gained weight, as the psychological feelings of restriction they imposed on themselves drove them to eat more.

Weight control does not have to mean that you can never have the foods you enjoy, but it does mean that at some point you are going to have to become a little stricter with yourself, even if it is just to achieve the initial drop in weight that is highly motivating. It is worth committing to going hard with your behaviour changes right from the start. You need to give yourself the time and space to focus fully on your goal for a couple of weeks at least. It takes this amount of time to achieve consistent fat loss and to start consolidating the lifestyle changes that will support you in achieving your fat-loss goals over the weeks or months required to lose 5, 10 or more kilos.

Those who are especially experienced with a cycle of being off and on a diet will be all too familiar with the process of beginning a new program with the best of intentions only to become derailed or distracted very quickly, leaving it null and void, before sometime down the line starting over again. To avoid falling into this same unsatisfying cycle, the key is to commit fully for a period of time, so you begin to see results from get-go, which in turn fuels the motivation to keep going.

In practical terms this means clearing your diary for a couple of weeks, so you do not find yourself in situations where others are indulging in large quantities of calorie-dense food. It means removing all tempting foods at home and saying no to tempting treats and alcohol when you would usually indulge. It means going to bed earlier, so you get up earlier to exercise, and it means fully committing to your balanced meal plan rather than taking the parts of the plan you like and ignoring the rest. It basically means being honest with yourself. It means withdrawing permission to eat poor quality food and to skip your exercise and still expect to lose weight because you are 'trying'.

4. Focus on YOU and your needs

No matter who you talk to about food and diets, everyone has an opinion – your neighbour lost weight by cutting carbs, your best friend wants you to join Weight Watchers with her, and your sister swears that ordering meals online has changed her life. There is always a new fad or program and the seasoned weight-loss adherent has tried them all. They are constantly open to new programs, none of which seem to work long term.

Individuals who are truly ready to commit to managing their weight are able to ignore the constant white noise relating to fad diets and weight-loss promotions, and instead turn their concentration towards what they personally need to do to reach a healthy weight and maintain it. They are able to hold focus on their own goals and plan, no matter what is going on around them, and feel no reason to justify their choices or decisions to others.

Every single person has a different genetic makeup, so what works for one person to manage their weight may be quite different for someone else. Some people may appear to be 'genetically blessed' and not have to do much, but in our experience this is rare. Most people have to work pretty hard to control their weight even if they do not openly admit it. If you are unsure of the changes that would be helpful for you individually, this is where a consultation with a dietitian or qualified personal trainer may help. They can assist you in identifying areas in your life that need focus and in making adjustments to help you reach your goals.

The truth is, we never know what other people do behind closed doors and, to be honest, we should not care. Concentrating solely on ourselves and what we need to do to look and be at our best is one of the easiest ways to take control of our bodies and, ultimately, our long-term health.

SIGNS YOU ARE TRULY COMMITTED TO YOUR NEW HEALTH PLAN

- You have cleared your calendar as much as possible to keep your healthy approach on track.
- You have shared your goals with family members and friends so they can support you.
- You have cleared the house of tempting treats and foods you know you should not be eating.
- You have created an exercise schedule and put it into your diary.
- You have shopped and planned your healthy meals and snacks.

It's 'easy for some'

Among the women we work with who want to lose weight, we often hear expressions of resentment that it is 'not fair' that they seem to have to work so much harder than others when it comes to weight control. While it is true that we're each working with our own unique bodies, metabolisms and genetics, there is no 'easy fix' for any of us. It's a matter of learning to understand what does and doesn't work for our body and focusing our attention on that.

Yes, there are people who are naturally slim who may need to work a lot less at proactively controlling their weight. There are also some people who struggle to carry enough weight to stay healthy. At various times in our lives we may personally find it 'easier' or 'harder' to manage our weight, depending on our current health and circumstances. Rather than wasting precious time and energy worrying over this inequity, accept that it is one of the realities of our existence and turn your attention to getting the best results for you based on where you're at in this moment.

Let's not forget, much of what we believe to be true is often based on assumptions. In many cases we see a very small proportion of someone's daily habits and behaviours. While some people may 'appear' to control their weight effortlessly, or 'appear' to be working very hard at weight control yet not getting anywhere, you only see parts of their day and therefore don't really know if this is the case. They may be up at 4 am exercising for an hour every day, they may eat very differently at home, or they may have private health issues. Honestly, unless you observe it for yourself, you won't know. We simply cannot assume we know or understand anyone else's reality.

As practising dietitians we see many hundreds of women, and the vast majority must work diligently to keep their weight under control. In fact, the science shows us those individuals who successfully maintain their weight follow 3 basic principles: they move a lot, exercise regularly and are consciously aware of their food choices on a daily basis.[14] Once you accept these behaviours into your own daily approach, you'll free up time and energy and banish resentment to focus on what you can actively do to keep your body healthy.

The good news is that we have ways to make this easier. And the first step is: creating a system! That's what we'll now look at in Chapter 3. One of the best ways to maintain positive habits is to establish systems at home and at work that help us choose the healthy lifestyle option by default. Let's look at how to create your own positive systems for success.

CHAPTER 3

SUCCESS IS
A SYSTEM

Most people think that knowledge is crucial. But when it comes to weight control and nutrition, planning is the key to success. Let's be honest: most of us know what we should (or should not) be eating – we know that fruits and vegetables are good, and we know that fried food is not so good. We know that chocolate is high in calories, and we know that eating less of it can help us lose weight. Knowledge is not the issue; rather, successful weight control is about creating environments around us that support healthy lifestyle choices, so they become the easy or default option.

It's the individual daily decisions that add up to give you positive lifestyle change, and you can enhance the impact of these decisions when you bring planning into the equation. In our busy, overscheduled lives, many of us don't have the systems in place to keep our exercise and dietary goals on track. However, pre-planning a routine action for each situation we might face – what to eat and and how to fit in our exercise – helps us foresee any barriers and complexities that might throw us off track, so we can put contingencies in place.

The simple act of planning helps to ensure that we are not caught off guard without the healthy foods we need to eat well. It helps to facilitate exercise compliance and it helps to predict occasions in which it will be difficult to eat well or exercise, so we can make alternative plans rather than falling victim to our environment or situation. Basically, planning helps us to remain in control and regulate our own health behaviours so that they are not impacted by external variables outside our control.

Goal setting is important, but without a solid system and implementation plan, a goal is just a dream. A solid system sets you up for success because it automates many of the steps that will take you forward. It also gives you a template or formula you can continue to change and modify over time to keep achieving new goals for yourself.

Meet Laura: a people-pleaser putting everyone else first

Laura, a 39-year-old mum of 3, was caught in the perpetual motion of attending to her family's needs, and as a result, was neglecting her own health. With a goal to lose 5 to 7 kilograms, increase her energy levels and reintegrate exercise into her life, when Laura came for a dietitian consultation and nutrition coaching, the approach quickly became about implementing new systems that would prioritise her wellbeing amid the demands of motherhood.

Laura's existing daily routine was a testament to her self-sacrificing nature. Breakfast was often skipped as she busied herself with packing her kids' lunches and ushering them out the door. Her mornings ran on autopilot, fuelled by multiple coffees with full-cream milk and sugar, while lunch was makeshift and on the go: sushi, a sausage roll or a large wrap. Often she'd skip it altogether and get by purely on snacks: nut bars, rice crackers and hummus, nuts and fruit or her kids' biscuits and chips. Dinner was the only somewhat balanced meal of the day, though it catered to her family's preferences for high-fat proteins, heavy carb-based dishes and minimal vegetables, with no room for her own needs.

Feeling sluggish and overwhelmed, Laura had realised that her approach to meals and exercise was unsustainable. She was cooking multiple dinners each night to appease her fussy eaters and found no time to focus on her own dietary needs. Grocery shopping had become a battleground, with her children's pleas for unhealthy snacks often winning over her better judgment (or patience!).

With guidance and support, Laura set about creating a structured system that would streamline her approach to nutrition and exercise. She started by engaging her family in the process. Her husband agreed to take on the kids' morning routine 3 times a week, allowing Laura to carve out time for exercise. Her mother-in-law's weekend visits became an opportunity for Laura to plan her meals and complete her grocery shopping in peace.

To tackle the issue of cooking multiple meals, Laura introduced deconstructed dinners. This approach allowed each family member to customise their plate, while Laura could focus on her own portion control and nutrient balance. She began meal prepping lean proteins for herself, ensuring she had quick and healthy options ready to go, and avoiding the temptation of high-calorie family favourites like sausages and crumbed chicken, which didn't align with her fat-loss goals.

To avoid skipping meals, Laura adopted the habit of packing her own lunchbox while preparing her kids' lunches. This simple act ensured she had access to healthy food throughout the day, reducing her reliance on snacks and takeaway. She also made a conscious effort to prepare her breakfast the night before, swapping her early-morning coffees for a more balanced start to the day.

To further support her weight-loss journey, Laura and her husband implemented 'family movement Sundays', encouraging active play and exercise for the whole family. This weekly routine not only provided Laura with a consistent opportunity to work out but also instilled the value of health and fitness in her children.

The impact of these new systems was profound. In just 12 weeks, Laura achieved a weight loss of 7.5 kilograms and dropped nearly two dress sizes. Her energy levels soared, and she found an increased strength and cardiovascular stamina for regular workouts. Her digestion improved significantly, thanks to the increased fibre and better quality choices in her diet, and she experienced fewer cravings and reduced menstrual discomfort each month. Her sleep quality improved and she felt more rested and alert throughout the day.

By implementing these strategic changes, Laura transformed her health and lifestyle. The structured approach to meal prep, exercise and family involvement not only facilitated her weight loss but also empowered her to maintain these healthy habits long term. With her newfound knowledge and systems in place, Laura confidently stepped into a healthier future for herself and her family.

The power of planning

When it comes to weight-related goals, planning is powerful. In fact, individuals who take the time to plan their exercise and food intake in advance have been shown to double their weight-loss outcomes compared to non-planners.[15]

The people who appear to achieve, keep fit and have it all together are not magically 'better' than anyone else. In this frantic life, it's often simply that they are more organised and this is especially true when it comes to eating and exercise. If the healthy food you need to eat well is not readily available, it is going to be pretty hard to eat it. If the training sessions are not booked in, clearing room in your busy schedule gets that much harder, and if you get home at 10 pm and there is no dinner, it is highly likely you will grab something quick and less nutritious than a proper meal, such as toast, cereal or yoghurt.

Planning is such a simple concept, yet so powerful. The key is taking the active steps to make time to do it – every day, every week, every month and every year. Otherwise, over time, life will simply take over and you will again find yourself out of routine, out of control and not directing your own food and exercise behaviours.

For example, you might look ahead to the weekly weather forecast and see rain ahead, so you know you will need to replace walking outside with another form of exercise. Or, if you check your diary in advance and see you have a work conference, you could organise to take food with you so you are not left reliant upon often less-than-nutritious conference catering.

Setting aside an hour or so each week to plan out a couple of meals, shop ahead, prepare a meal or two and schedule your training is such a simple strategy and often the only thing that stands between us being on track or not with our food, our training and our weight.

Make it a habit

Contrary to popular belief, it is not strict diet regimes or hours and hours spent at the gym that predict weight control. In fact, it has been shown that what is much more powerful when it comes to losing weight and keeping it off are the healthy lifestyle habits that underpin our daily routine.[16]

The key to building good habits – small repeatable behaviours – is in ensuring they fit into your lifestyle, are sustainable, and you enjoy them, as then you are more likely to keep going rather than give up after a few days or weeks because it is either too hard or you simply don't like doing it. Habits are formed when we repeat a behaviour over time until it becomes automatic.

In the case of diet and exercise, there are several small but powerful habits that will go a long way in building a strong foundation for weight control. When resetting your lifestyle, a good place to start is with building a strong, healthy eating platform. Once these habits become more firmly entrenched, you can start to examine other more personal habits that will transform your current regime into one of optimal health and wellbeing.

For example, a classic habitual behaviour is buying a coffee on the way to work. Each day, at 8 am, we stop at the café and order a coffee, and often, a slice of banana bread. Although in our new health approach we may have decided to no longer buy the banana bread, if the two purchases have typically gone hand in hand, their familiar association makes it more likely to happen. If your new goal is to eat less banana bread, then breaking the connection can help – perhaps stop buying the coffee, or at least buy it somewhere else until you have established a new habit.

Your 5 core healthy habits

1. Eat more vegetables

If you apply your focus to significantly increasing your vegetable intake, simply by making sure that you include at least 1 to 2 serves of vegetables or salad each and every time you eat, not only will your overall nutritional intake be improved, but your overall calorie intake will be reduced without you even noticing. We'll come back to this habit in a big way in Chapter 8!

2. Prioritise movement

Individuals who have lost significant amounts of weight and kept it off tend to exercise a lot. Though specifics vary according to age and health conditions, Australian government guidelines advise that adults under 65 should be active on most (preferably all) days and, as health permits, include both moderate (for example, walking, swimming) and vigorous exercise (for example, jogging, fast cycling) as well as muscle-strengthening activities.[17] If your ultimate goal is to be healthy and in control of your weight long term, the sooner you start to factor in some exercise as part of your daily routine, the better.

3. Take time to plan

Planning is the key to dietary success as it helps us have healthy foods, ensuring we can eat well most of the time. This means making it a priority each week to shop, plan meals and snacks in advance, and prepare your snacks and meals a day ahead, so you don't get caught without the healthy foods on hand that you need to keep your calorie intake under control.

4. Cook more at home

Generally, as soon as we buy food away from the home (even if it is a 'healthier' option), we tend to consume a higher number of calories. Restaurant, café and food court meals are typically packed full of extra fats and calories and can often be served in larger portion sizes than might suit your plan. For this reason, committing to more food prep at home will go a long way towards keeping your calorie intake controlled.

5. Focus on consistency

One of the most common traits of serial dieters is that they are either 'on' or 'off' a program at any one time. On the other hand, individuals who manage to keep their weight stable have been shown to keep their diet consistent most of the time.[18] Sure, they may enjoy a meal off-plan occasionally, or a piece of cake at a party, but most of the time they maintain a healthy, balanced approach to eating that's free of fad diets, routine overeating or entire days of over-indulgence.

How to shift unhelpful habits

HABIT THAT DOESN'T SERVE YOU	HEALTHIER HABIT
Overeating after work	Snacking on an apple on the way home so you're not hungry when arriving home.
Eating the kids' leftovers	Chewing some gum while cleaning up so you are not tempted to mindlessly eat.
Pouring a glass of wine as soon as you get home	Pouring a glass of sparkling water as soon as you walk in the door.
Overeating after dinner	Enjoying a 100-calorie after-dinner treat, then brushing your teeth.
Eating too much at dinner	Serving up an appropriate portion, then immediately boxing up leftovers, as it is harder to overeat food that is not in front of you.
Inspired by these examples, create your own list of habits to shift	

Let's talk about . . . the people around you

A powerful influence on what we eat and when – beyond will-power, motivation or even following a plan – is the people we spend time with and the environments in which we live. Human beings are heavily influenced by those around them, so to a large degree we end up eating and exercising like those we're close to. As the 32-year-long Framingham Heart Study determined, 'obesity appears to spread through social ties'.[19]

This means that if your goal is to eat well and exercise most of the time, it's wise to consider what happens when you spend a lot of time with friends, family or even at work. This doesn't need to mean reducing the time spent with those people – instead, it's about clearly communicating your goals and intentions to them and requesting that they support you to achieve them.

Your partner

Partners are notorious for playing a lead role in sabotaging their better half's diet, especially when they themselves are not wanting to make the healthy choices. You need to be strong with this one and it may be wise to separate your personal eating and exercise habits from your partner's, even preparing separate meals if you have to. It also helps to be honest with them. Point out that bringing home chocolates and treats or tempting you with alcohol is undermining your efforts.

Your family

The powerful programming effects of our early experiences with food can mean that we instantly return to childhood with our food habits when we are in the presence of family. There are also the 'feeders' who routinely offer you large volumes of delicious home-cooked, heavy foods that feel literally impossible to refuse. Where possible say no, especially to empty calorie foods such as snacks, lollies and chocolates. At those times when consuming some of the extra food is inevitable, focus on portion control and bulking up your plate with extra veggies and salad where you can.

Your mother

For women in particular, our relationship with food is closely tied to the relationship we have with our mothers and what they taught us, including their own connection to food. It is not uncommon to hear stories of supposedly well-meaning mothers letting their daughters know they have gained weight while continuing to feed them tempting treats. Indeed, this can be a very challenging relationship.

Depending on your circumstances, you may be able to have an honest chat with your mum and specifically ask her not to cook, buy and offer you the exact foods you are trying to avoid. If this kind of direct conversation is not for you, try replacing meals at her place with walks or coffee catch-ups, or invite her to your home instead, where you're more able to remain in control of your food options.

Your in-laws

Our long-term partner and their relatives will inevitably impact our habits, thoughts and behaviours over time, too. Sometimes it can be harder to say no to our in-laws than our own family, especially in the early stages of a relationship. If your mother-in-law wants you to eat, she will do everything in her power to make it hard not to! In social situations where a larger number of people are present it is much easier to avoid or divert attention, but this gets harder in smaller gatherings. When only a couple of you are being served, the easiest way to manage the situation is to accept the food on offer, but then to eat slowly and mindfully to consume only as much food as you wish. Ask for your partner's support, too – either to act as a buffer or, if they're onboard, to help you finish the higher calorie meals and desserts that you are trying to avoid.

Your kids

As parents we are often guilty of forgetting to take care of ourselves. When we're busy and tired, often our diet becomes a mix of kids' food and leftovers as well as their sugary drinks and treats. Then there are the child-friendly restaurant and takeaway meals, which tend to be high-carb and high-fat, that we end up eating, too. The easiest way to avoid these blowouts is by satisfying your nutritional needs first. While it may go against the grain, choosing your cuisine first, packing your own snacks and eating your breakfast before the kids are some of the best ways to avoid eating highly processed kids' food too frequently. Keep in mind, though, such foods are generally not good options for your kids either, so if you can make over the whole family's eating habits to be healthier, everyone will benefit.

Your friends

Put most simply, if your friends regularly exercise and make healthy meal choices when eating out, you are far more likely to keep your weight under control than if your friends make poor food choices, don't move much and carry extra weight. Most commonly, friends can consciously or unconsciously play a 'feeder' role, in which they encourage you to eat foods you may not really want. It is also common for time spent with friends to have a food focus – for example, catching up over drinks or dinner – so this can take some navigating.

To stay on track, it's important to differentiate between special occasions and routine get-togethers, to avoid the trap of always consuming wine or desserts if your catch-ups are frequent. For this reason, it is important to be honest and transparent with those closest to you and be confident to stand up for yourself and say when you are keen for a heathier option – choosing a clean-eating restaurant, or catching up for a walk and coffee rather than a sit-down brunch.

Your colleagues

The fact that so many of us spend so many hours each week at work can be a disaster when it comes to our diets, especially if our workplaces are not all that healthy. The combination of the fundraising chocolates, regular birthday cakes, unhealthy vending machines and office feeders can really derail our plan when it comes to our overall calorie intake. Avoid overeating at the office by planning ahead and taking your food where you can, and get used to saying no to the incessant feeders and bakers.

NOTES FROM THE NUTRITION COUCH
HOW TO MOVE FROM A FIXED TO A GROWTH MINDSET

The language we use can unlock success in the long term. If you think making a change in your life is going to be challenging, chances are it's going to feel that way, too. Instead of counting yourself out before you even begin, be kind to yourself and concentrate on possible solutions rather than what you think will stop you from being successful.

- Fixed mindset: 'I'm too busy to eat healthy, I have young kids and no time for myself. There's no point cooking a healthy meal this week, I'll just get something convenient because I don't have the energy.'
- Growth mindset: 'I want to work with the time I have to make healthy choices. To do this I'm going to sit down and work out how I can fit in cooking a healthy meal for myself this week. I will look up some time-effective recipes that contain the nutrients I need for the week.'

If it feels like a big jump between a fixed and a growth mindset, aim to start small. Remain action focused. Think about any possible opportunities you have in your schedule to work towards your health and wellbeing goals.

24 May 2023[20]

Set yourself up for success

If you're serious about getting the results you want for your body, you need to set yourself up for success by ensuring that your regular environments – be that home, work or other people's houses – match your goals. When we're tired after a long day, we often default back to easy options, so if your environment doesn't encourage easy, healthy choices, you're more likely to go against yourself.

Start by cleaning out your fridge and pantry and giving away any unhealthy, high-calorie and highly processed foods you know are not aligned with the goals you have for your body. Rearrange your fridge and pantry so that healthy food is at eye level and easily accessible. To reduce daily temptation, keep treats out of sight and store them in a box or container with a lid.

Once you have an environment that supports your goals, you need to recruit your loved ones to support you. As we've touched on, being clear and communicating your goals to friends and family is really important if you want to succeed in the long term. You'll find great strength in your support system and their encouragement, especially when your own motivation or willpower wanes, or you experience a setback.

You may gain further support in other ways – for instance, joining a group-exercise program or online health forum, or hiring a coach for accountability. Involving other people in our health journey is important as they can offer us a fresh perspective. Often we struggle to see the things that may be right in front of us or holding us back. Improving our relationship with food takes trial and error and having a support network to bounce ideas off and remind us of our long-term goals can be incredibly useful.

Seeing your goals multiple times a day is often very helpful for sustained success. If you're someone who thrives off quotes and motivational slogans, get out a pen and paper and write your goals down and pin them up in the kitchen somewhere visible. Setting training or exercise goals and checking them off can also bolster motivation. Tracking these through various online platforms can add a fun element of friendly competition.

When it comes to getting started and setting yourself up for success, planning ahead and staying organised is paramount. To prevent impulse eating and poor food choices, plan your meals in advance and use this to write a shopping list before you go to the supermarket. This way you'll be less likely to impulse buy at the shops, less likely to waste food, and more likely to eat well. It also means you'll have the ingredients you need to prepare nourishing meals without needing to rush back to the supermarket multiple times a week, which in itself can derail your intentions to eat well.

Once you have your plan for nourishing meals, set aside some time to do a little meal prep. You can prep every meal for the next 3 days, or just focus on breakfasts for a few days, or perhaps just prep the protein portion of your meal. A little goes a long way. Preparing food ahead will save you time during the week and increases the likelihood that you'll eat well after a long, hard day. It's worth doing if you can make the time in advance.

If you're not a fan of eating complete meals cooked ahead of time, focus on preparing healthy snacks. Cut up vegetable sticks such as carrot and celery and place them in a jar of water in the fridge so they stay crisp for the week. Boil some eggs in advance for a quick and easy snack. Make some mini savoury muffins, so instead of reaching for the block of chocolate, you can enjoy a homemade savoury snack instead.

Create your own system that's suited to you and your life. Building upon your new healthy eating mindset from Chapter 1 and the commitment you developed in Chapter 2, you're well on your way to success.

SYSTEMS FOR SUCCESS

Here are our top hacks for a successful system when it comes to health and weight loss:

- Clean out your cupboards and fridge regularly.
- Plan your meals ahead and prepare food in advance.
- Shop with a grocery list and never shop hungry.
- Cook in bulk so you have healthy leftovers for lunch and freezer meals.
- Only buy foods you truly love, and fewer of them if they don't support your goals.
- Buy smaller-sized treat portions, like 'mini' or 'lunchbox' or kids' varieties.
- Keep temptation foods out of sight and store them in a box with a lid.
- Practise mindful eating – slow down and savour each mouthful.
- Place healthy foods at eye level in the fridge/pantry.
- Pack your lunch the night before.
- Consistently support your health goals, even on weekends.

- Keep indulgences to small occasional treats or single meals, not a full day.
- Be kind to yourself and understand it's a journey that doesn't have to be perfect.
- Create a support system of loved ones, community and professionals.
- Actively schedule time for planning ahead each week, to keep you on track.

Enjoy the process

Congratulations on completing Reset. Creating this platform for real change may be the fundamental difference between your diets of the past and long-lasting success moving forward. Across our busy lives, we rarely take time out to reflect and genuinely consider what we want, what is holding us back from getting there, and what changes we can make to take us closer to the goals we have for ourselves. Reset has encouraged you to take this time to understand your underlying motivations, identify the areas of your lifestyle that need work, and plan systems in your life to help you reach your goals. You have paved the way to your own healthy eating foundation. Now, let's build on that in Nourish.

PART 2

NOURISH

NOW,
LET'S NOURISH

Now that we have reset our thinking around food, dieting and good health, let's turn our attention to practical ways to support this new mindset. This next phase, Nourish, focuses on good quality nutrition. So many of the women we see struggle to understand how to strike a balance between optimising nutrient intake and keeping their weight under control. They tend to overeat yet lack the key nutrients they need to feel, look and perform at their best. Because of this, they often find themselves carrying more weight than they'd like, then fall into the diet cycle, which continues to derail their attempts to build an optimal nutrition platform.

For some of us, all we've really known is what it's like to be 'on' or 'off' a diet. We've never really known the foundations of a nutritionally balanced approach to eating or how to eat to nourish and fuel the body. Given the huge array of diets and often-conflicting nutrition science available on the internet, this is not surprising. Even if we want to follow 'best practice' it's often difficult to know what that is. With social media flourishing, it seems like every second person is an 'expert' in some type of nutrition, selling their way as the best way. But until you understand the basic scientific principles of nutrition so you can apply them to your personal goals and individual body and lifestyle, you will generally struggle with trying to adopt someone else's approach and make it work for you.

Getting it right starts by creating a personalised approach founded on science-based nutrition fundamentals. Unfortunately these have not always been taught or communicated in a clear way. For this reason, the Nourish phase focuses on explaining, in easy-to-understand terms, sound nutrition principles. Throughout, we'll answer common questions on nutrition and provide useful and practical tips on how to implement good habits into your daily routine. We'll cover all the basics and clear up the confusion to give you a solid foundation upon which to build your own nutrition best practice.

SIGNS YOU NEED TO GET BETTER AT NOURISHING YOUR BODY

- You do not know what to eat and when.
- You think you eat 'healthy' but do not feel great.
- You do not plan your meals and snacks in advance.
- You always find yourself eating on the run.
- You skip meals even when you don't mean to.
- You are always hungry and rarely satisfied.
- You often crave sugar.
- You eat the same things all the time.
- You have constant digestive issues.
- You know you are not eating enough fresh food.
- You often eat out and never know what to order or choose to be healthy.
- You often feel like you're on an energy rollercoaster, with a few big slumps in the day.

Nourish – boost your everyday power

One of the biggest issues of nutrition and diet, particularly with regards to weight loss, is that few of us really know what we are doing. Every time another 'expert' appears in the media we are swayed towards their latest and greatest secret for diet success and then, a few weeks later when it hasn't worked, we are left feeling even more confused and frustrated than when we started.

Whether you choose to go low carb, high protein, calorie count or adopt a mix of dietary approaches, the most important thing when it comes to losing weight and controlling it long term is to *understand* what you are doing. If you do not understand the fundamental principles of weight management, you will always have to rely on someone else's plan to know what you should be eating. But if you're aware of sound nutritional practices and know why they work, such as including protein each time you eat to keep you less hungry between meals, or how vegetables or salad help to boost your fibre intake and will help you to feel full, you will be able to put these dietary practices into daily action with confidence. The more you know, the more you can personally direct your own successful approach to weight management.

Adding to the knowledge we gained in the Reset phase, Nourish is founded on 3 core principles to help you build sustained strength and energy for a long and healthy life:

1. Nourish for energy
2. Nourish for strength
3. Nourish for optimal health

Why are these topics so important? Firstly, because as part of our efforts to ditch diet culture we want to turn your attention away from calorie counting and towards nourishing your body. Knowing what to eat and when has a huge impact on our energy levels, which in turn affect our lives, our behaviours and decisions, our performance – and even our relationships. Many of us are letting outside forces dictate our energy levels instead of realising we can harness them ourselves through simple daily choices about what we eat and drink, and when.

Secondly, because too many women underestimate how significantly the type of food they're eating affects both their short-term performance and long-term health. When clients come to us, we'll commonly see that the major food groups in their diet are out of balance and are not supporting their health, energy and lifestyle goals. They're fuelling with the wrong types of carbohydrates and fats, while protein and fibre feature too little in their diet. Knowing how to redress this imbalance is the key to unlocking a whole host of benefits for your body, now and into the future.

And lastly, because a happy gut helps with a happy life. As scientists have come to better understand, our gut plays a central role in how our bodies feel and function, affecting many things such as mood, cognition, sleep and mental health.[21] Often we find that improving our gut health can have a positive impact on a host of other issues too. If we know how to love our gut, it will love us back. And improving our gut microbiome starts with what we eat.

CHAPTER 4

NOURISH FOR ENERGY

Too often, our days are punctuated by energy slumps that leave us reaching for the nearest caffeine fix or sweet hit, a temporary solution that can lead us into a vicious cycle of erratic blood sugar levels and disrupted sleep. Until we've been taught, we can be quite oblivious to the impact of our food choices throughout the day on how alert or sluggish we feel, often eating with good intentions that have an unintentionally negative domino effect. We've all felt the grip of mid-afternoon cravings, a telltale sign of our body's search for a quick energy boost!

But here's the truth: we have far more control over our energy than we realise. One of the greatest benefits of understanding good nutrition is learning how to balance our energy cycle. This means peeling back the layers of fatigue, understanding the intricate dance of blood sugar, insulin, sleep, caffeine and hormones, and learning how to nourish ourselves well to create sustained energy that carries us through our day.

Our energy is what powers our whole lives, allowing us to do the things that matter to us: playing with our kids, working with clarity and focus, keeping active, travelling to new places, taking care of relatives. So, let's get wise to what's happening inside our bodies so we can bring our most dynamic, vibrant selves to it all.

Food as energy

'Energy' can be described in many ways: in terms of how we are feeling, our internal get-up-and-go, and our ability to respond to what's going on around us. A large part of our energy is generated by the food we eat. Many of us often don't realise just how much the way we *feel* is impacted by what we eat.

In food terms, energy refers to the molecules produced after we consume food, and how they are utilised by the body to fuel the muscles and the brain. Different types of food produce different amounts of energy, and this is where the concept of calories is relevant. The human body requires a certain number of calories to function, and each day we get these required calories (and often more) from the food we eat. Although in Australia kilojoules are the standard measure, discussions around food energy are more commonly presented using calories, so we will use this term moving forward.

Calories are not the devil

For some of us, the mere mention of the word calorie is enough to ignite a lot of stress and anxiety. But this shouldn't be the case; calories are simply a unit measure of energy. While calories are commonly associated with 'counting' and weight loss, the reality is they are just a tool to help us understand our energy demands.

We all need calories, but since different foods are loaded with different types of energy and nutrient value, it's important to understand a food's breakdown. Focusing on the quality of the calories we choose, as well as understanding where extra calories can slip into our daily food choices, can make a big difference when it comes to health and weight control. If you see kilojoules written on a nutrition label, simply divide them by roughly 4.2 to get the calorie amount.

How many calories do I need?

Every single person has a different calorie requirement to survive and our daily energy requirements are further affected by the effort we expend; lying around obviously uses far less energy than running a marathon. Our 'basal metabolic rate' (BMR) is the minimum energy/calorie intake we need to keep our bodily organs functioning while we are at rest; to breathe, pump blood, et cetera. To simply stay alive, the average adult requires anywhere between 1200 and 2000 calories a day. This does not allow for any additional energy required for digestion, moving about and undertaking daily tasks, not to mention higher energy activities such as working out, running around after others, or working in a high-stress job.

As such, each person's daily calorie requirement is different. On average, a small female's minimum energy requirement falls between 1200 and 1600 calories a day. Calorie requirements should be adjusted according to exercise requirements and weight-loss goals. The best way to determine your calorie requirement is to calculate your BMR and add any additional calorie requirements based on your lifestyle and activities. Calorie-restricted diets will generally encourage a reduction in calorie intake on your calculated daily requirement by around 300 to 500 calories a day.

It's also important to consider that just as the number of calories we need can vary each day, so too can our appetite. Our hormones, energy output and lifestyle can all affect our food intake, so on some days you may feel full and satisfied after sticking to your eating plan, while on others you may be hungrier and need more. Eating for special occasions will also spike your calorie intake. And this is all fine – perfectly normal and to be expected. As we learnt in Reset, the best approach is to apply our 'balanced eating' mindset and not get so hung up on one day or one meal, but rather consider our overall approach. What determines our weight is maintaining the right balance of calories over time; how they fluctuate on daily basis is less important.

A ROUGH GUIDE ONLY

An important thing to know about calories is that wherever they are listed, they should be used as a guideline only. If used to determine your daily calorie requirements or analyse the calorie load of foods, the calories listed on common apps and calculators are not an absolute reference. Generally speaking, on these apps and devices the calories listed may be inaccurate by as much as 20 per cent. That's why we recommend referring to calories as a rough guide rather than aiming for strict compliance. If you think about calories and calculators in this way, you are more likely to use them to your advantage.

Metabolism

Put simply, metabolism is the body's means of converting food to energy to drive all the processes our body undertakes to stay alive – such things as cardiac output, respiration, body temperature, protein synthesis and muscle function, as well as the metabolic function itself and energy storage. When more energy is consumed than is needed for metabolism and physical activity, the excess is stored, primarily as adipose tissue (body fat).

As described above, our basal metabolic rate, or BMR, is the minimum calories (food/fuel) our body needs to generate the energy we require to survive. Roughly 75 per cent of this daily calorie requirement is determined by body shape and size. People with greater amounts of muscle mass need more calories than smaller individuals. The remaining 25 per cent is dependent on your activity levels and on what kind of foods you eat and how often.

Typically, as we age we need fewer calories, due to less activity and a general loss in muscle mass that adults experience throughout their late thirties, forties and beyond. It becomes harder to prevent weight gain as we age because the average adult will see a gradual reduction in muscle mass, the type of tissue in the body that actively burns calories.

For this reason, making a concerted effort to eat and exercise in a way that helps to optimise your metabolism and keep the body burning fuel efficiently is a smart way to help avoid gradually increasing your weight each year. As protein requires slightly more calories to burn than fat or carbohydrate, protein-rich foods like meat, eggs or dairy help to support small increases in metabolic rate.

SIMPLE AND SCIENCE-BACKED WAYS TO INCREASE YOUR METABOLIC RATE

Ensure you are eating enough protein throughout the day	Protein supports our muscle mass and as muscle is a metabolically active tissue, the more you have, the better your metabolism will be. If you're not eating enough protein, you're likely to be losing muscle mass, which can decrease your metabolism over time.
Include weight training in your exercise program	Weight training a few times a week can help to build and retain muscle and as muscle is a metabolically active tissue, the more you have, the better your metabolism will be.
Keep mixing things up	Your body gets used to doing the same thing and gets more efficient at it over time, so needs less energy to perform the same task. Refrain from eating the same thing each day and change the timing and portions of your meals regularly, too, in order to boost your metabolism.
Change up your exercise	As above, the body gets used to doing the same thing and gets more efficient at it over time, so you need to ensure the type and length of your training is changed up every few months.

Eat enough calories – don't stay in a deficit for too long	The longer you spend in a calorie deficit, the more your body reduces your calorie expenditure, so if you're not losing/have plateaued in weight, reverse diet by strategically and slowly adding more calories to your diet until you have returned to eating at maintenance-level calories.

Macronutrients are the key

Often chronic dieters will jump straight to focusing their attention on overall calorie intake and energy expenditure. While a useful guide, this is a very simplistic approach to energy management and weight loss. Resetting this focus is a key part of our approach. We not only want to break the diet cycle, but more importantly, we want to teach you how to use nutrition to your advantage – which foods to eat when, in order to best support your health and weight goals over the long term.

Well before calorie counting, first and foremost it is critical to understand the role macronutrients play in our overall health and wellbeing, so this is our primary focus here in the Nourish phase. Once you understand how to work with macronutrients to best support your health, energy and strength goals then, in the Burn phase, we can turn our focus to how to fine tune calorie management and other smart strategies for weight loss and long-term weight management.

Food is made up of 4 energy-giving macronutrients – carbohydrates, proteins, fats and alcohol. The body breaks these nutritive components down through the metabolic process and uses them to generate energy which it uses as fuel to maintain the body's structure and keep it functioning. When more energy is consumed than is needed for metabolism and physical activity, the excess is stored, primarily as body fat. To determine our overall energy intake we add up the combined energy total of the macronutrients in our diet. But it's not as straightforward as it sounds because they each carry a different calorie load per gram:

- Carbohydrate – 4 calories (16.7 kJ) per gram
- Protein – 4 calories (16.7 kJ) per gram
- Fat – 9 calories (37.7 kJ) per gram
- Alcohol – 7 calories (29.3 kJ) per gram

Each food contains a different mix of these macronutrients in varying proportions. As such, foods tend to be grouped according to their dominant macronutrient. For example: red meat, chicken and fish contain both protein and fat but since their protein ratio is higher, they are generally referred to as protein-based foods. On the other hand, while bread, rice and pasta do contain small amounts of protein (some more than others) they are predominantly carbs, so are known as carbohydrate-based foods.

When determining what to eat and when, it's important to get the balance of macronutrients right. As each of them (apart from alcohol) plays an essential role in our diet, be very wary of any diet plan that encourages you to cut out any major food group entirely. While it's very general to state that each macronutrient performs a specific role, since their best work is done in combination, it is broadly accepted that among the many functions they perform each has a primary duty: carbs for energy and gut health, protein for strength and metabolic function, and essential fats for optimal brain and cellular function.

A NOTE ON ALCOHOL

As it provides energy that the body burns for fuel, alcohol is technically a macronutrient, but unlike the other 3 it is not essential for our survival. Our body identifies alcohol as a toxin, so burns it off first to protect our vital organs. Metabolised mainly by the liver, in normal functioning it takes around one hour to process one standard drink. If you are aiming for weight loss, alcohol adds non-essential calories to your diet, increasing the challenge of caloric reduction. Studies have found that when consumed, it is substituted for more nutrient-dense foods and stimulates the appetite for less healthy foods, which can lead to malnutrition and decreased performance and recovery – not to mention the effects of alcohol itself.[22]

Alcohol is a powerful diuretic, meaning that it increases urine output, which is why your head commonly hurts the morning after a few drinks. As the body is up to 60 per cent water, even just 1 to 2 per cent reductions in overall fluid levels in the body can have profound effects on how we look, feel and perform on a daily basis. Cells with a high turnover, like our skin, will respond almost instantly to dehydration, leaving us looking dull and listless. Alcohol also impairs our gut, contributing to IBS, diarrhoea or constipation, and abdominal discomfort.[23] And we all know that it impacts our ability to focus and concentrate.

Then, there is the way alcohol impacts our sleep. Many of us may turn to a drink or two to relax after a long day, and as a nervous system depressant, alcohol will feel like a sleep aid. However, the quality of our sleep is likely to be affected if we've had something to drink. Specifically, it appears that REM or restorative sleep is disrupted after alcohol consumption, which may explain why you feel especially tired and lethargic after a night on the drink. In addition, for those who snore or have diag-nosed sleep apnoea, as alcohol suppresses breathing, it is likely to make your sleep apnoea even worse.[24]

And beyond performance, there are of course much greater health issues linked to alcohol consumption: the risk of developing any of the several lifestyle diseases associated with high con-sumption of alcohol, including liver disease, pancreatitis, stroke and a number of types of cancer.

While there may be some general public health recommen-dations on alcohol consumption, the reality is that there is no 'safe' amount of alcohol we should consume and when it comes to health and risk of disease the less alcohol we consume overall, the better.[25]

Carbohydrates for energy

As this chapter is about nourishing for energy, let's turn our focus to carbohydrates. In today's diet culture, carbs are often the most demonised of the major food groups. But like any of the macro-nutrients, if you understand how they work, you can use them in the right proportions and at the right times, to your advantage.

Carbohydrates are found in foods in 3 different forms – sugars, starch and fibre – each of which vary in their nutritional values and effects on health. Sugars are 'simple carbohydrates' and while a good instant energy source, unless you are using them as a pre-workout fuelling option, you're generally better off eating 'complex carbohydrates' – foods containing starches and fibre. These break down more slowly, which is better for keeping blood sugar steady and will help keep you full for longer.

From an energy perspective, carbohydrate-based foods such as bread, rice, cereal, pasta, fruits and sugars are broken down to supply glucose molecules in the body – glucose being the primary fuel for the muscles and the brain. While other foods like proteins and fats can also be used for this, they require a more complicated process and the body has to work harder to perform it, whereas glucose from carbohydrates is far more readily accessible. As such, carbohydrate intake significantly impacts our overall energy balance, our weight loss or gain, and our daily experience of energy.

There's no doubt we need carbohydrates in our diet to help fuel our bodies and support our energy levels. But which carbs we eat and how we consume them can make all the difference between experiencing creeping weight gain and blood-glucose issues, versus having a steady level of energy and finding weight management easier.

Understanding blood glucose

To make the most of our energy and to better manage or lose weight, we really need to get clear on the impact of carbohydrates and glucose. Much of our daily experience of energy can be attributed to our blood glucose levels. They are regulated by several variables including how much and the type of carbohydrates we consume, when we consume them, how active we are, and what is going on with our hormones, especially the hormone insulin.

For a long time, the discussion around blood glucose and insulin has been focused almost exclusively on people with diabetes. But recent research is showing how important it is for *all* of us to be aware of what our blood-glucose levels are doing on a regular basis, as our bodies all use insulin to manage our blood-glucose levels and help keep them steady. This is important, as elevated blood glucose can contribute to a range of health complications including damage to our organs and nerves, and increased risk of diabetes, infections and heart problems.[26]

Use it, or store it

As our body digests carbohydrates, it breaks them down into simple sugars (including glucose) that are absorbed into the bloodstream. As glucose enters the bloodstream, our blood sugar rises – an increase often referred to as a 'spike' in blood glucose levels. Depending on several factors including the type of carbs eaten, when they're eaten and with what (fibre, fat, protein), and an individual's metabolism, this spike can be sharper or more gradual.

When our blood glucose rises, the pancreas responds. It secretes insulin, a hormone that helps cells throughout the body absorb glucose and use it for energy. Like a key unlocking the door, insulin facilitates the entry of glucose into the cells, which can either use the glucose for immediate energy needs or store it for later use as glycogen in the liver and muscles. In this way, insulin is a key regulator of both glucose and fat metabolism in the body.

When your insulin is working as it should, it helps your cells absorb any excess glucose from the carbohydrates you consume. When you're exercising you'll use most of the glucose immediately, but when you eat a mid-morning muffin sitting at your desk, you're not using much at all. So it's stashed away instead, primarily as body fat, to potentially be burned in the future.

This is all fine if you typically expend roughly as much energy as you take onboard. The trouble comes if you don't use it, but keep adding more to your stored energy instead. This is where over-consuming carbs poses a challenge for weight loss. If you're not using the glucose from the carbohydrates you eat, that excess blood sugar ends up being deposited in your body's fat tissues, which can ultimately contribute to weight gain.[27]

NOTES FROM THE NUTRITION COUCH
THE LOWDOWN ON LOW-SUGAR ALTERNATIVES

- In the supermarkets, low-sugar alternatives to treats like chocolate and baked goods are often highly processed and expensive.
- Consuming low-sugar products can lead to overconsumption because people perceive them as healthier, so they might consume more.
- Consider enjoying smaller portions of the 'real deal' rather than opting for low-sugar versions to ensure true satisfaction and enjoyment.
- Be cautious of the physiological impact of consuming large amounts of low-calorie, low-sugar products, as it may lead to gut distress.

18 June 2023[28]

Insulin resistance

The body is in balance when the amount of insulin matches the amount of carbohydrate consumed and the blood glucose levels are controlled. For some individuals, largely as a result of a genetic predisposition but commonly as a result of weight gain over time, insulin can stop working as efficiently as it should. This is known as insulin resistance, and it can have a significant effect on blood glucose levels.

In a person with insulin resistance, the cells in the body become less sensitive to the insulin circulating in the bloodstream. As a result, the normal amount of insulin is not enough to unlock the cell doors and facilitate glucose entry. To compensate and attempt to maintain normal blood-glucose levels, the pancreas produces more insulin. Over time, this excess demand on the pancreas can lead to its decreased ability to produce insulin, potentially leading to the development of prediabetes and type 2 diabetes if glucose levels become too high.[29]

For this reason, if you have noticed that you are having unusual shifts in energy through the day, are craving sweet foods and gaining weight, it may be worth not only paying attention to what your blood glucose levels are doing but also what your insulin levels are like. Consult your doctor to find out more about your personal blood glucose and insulin levels.

SIGNS YOU COULD HAVE ISSUES WITH GLUCOSE CONTROL

Glucose regulation issues have a strong genetic component, which means if there is a family history of type 2 diabetes, and you have any signs or symptoms such as fluctuating glucose levels, unexplained weight gain, a high waist measurement or extreme sweet cravings, it may be time to check in with your GP and have your glucose levels clinically assessed.

The blood sugar rollercoaster

Another problem with high glucose spikes are the significant drop in blood glucose that follow. After insulin has carried unused glucose away to store in our cells, the levels of glucose in our blood start to fall, setting off a new chain of events. That brain fog, difficulty focusing, tiredness or sudden mid-afternoon slump of energy you experience could well be traced back to the carb-heavy meal you ate for lunch. Feeling low in energy, naturally you feel like reaching for something sweet, as many of us do to get through the afternoon.

And it would seem to make sense that we should grab something sugary or dense in carbs to give us a lift – after all, this is what diabetics do to counter a blood sugar low. It works, to a point, immediately boosting our blood sugar. Fine if you're managing diabetes, but not so great if you're just trying to juggle a regular day. That instant boost in blood sugar delivers an equally strong blood sugar crash to follow, which generally leaves us feeling even worse than we did before. We become so used to riding this blood sugar rollercoaster each day that we don't realise the turbulence we're putting our bodies through.

The good news is that as soon as we're aware of this cycle, we have the choice to step off the rollercoaster. With each new day we can decide not to step onto it in the first place, and nourish our bodies with greater wisdom. We can put ourselves back in control when we're feeling depleted or unstable in energy and gaining weight that we're desperate to keep off. Let's talk about how.

SLOW AND STEADY WINS THE RACE

Blood glucose levels are best controlled when we consume balanced meals containing lean protein, good quality fats, and salad and vegetables along with good quality carbohydrates such as wholegrains, starchy vegetables and legumes. This combination works together to release glucose into the bloodstream more slowly after eating, reducing peaks and drops in blood sugar levels.

Eating balanced meals slows digestion and ensures we feel both full and satisfied enough that we can comfortably go 3 to 4 hours between meals. This extended break from eating is ideal for blood glucose control as it gives our blood glucose levels a chance to return to baseline levels.

Unfortunately, few of us eat this way. Instead we tend to fill our days with small intakes of processed carbohydrates drip-fed into the body every hour or two: snacks, milk-based coffees, biscuits, crackers, unbalanced meals grabbed on the run, and sweet drinks such as coconut water and juices. Such high-carb foods send blood glucose levels soaring and the constant snacking interrupts prolonged periods without food, which are helpful for stabilising blood glucose levels.

From an energy perspective, this style of eating often means we tend to eat too much, rarely feel truly hungry and are constantly driving our blood glucose levels up and down. If you always feel tired, crave sweet treats and know your energy regulation is not at its best, it is time to take a closer look at how and what you are eating.

Meet Bridget: a low-carb under-eater 💼

Bridget's corporate life was dedicated to the pursuit of success, paralleled by her dedication to CrossFit. At 42, her goals were laser-focused: she wanted to dominate in her CrossFit sessions, trim down her body fat by 2 to 3 kilograms, and have sustained energy throughout the day.

Her dietary routine was a low-carb, low-fat regime. She began every day at the gym training on an empty stomach, not eating until hours after her workout had finished. Lunch and dinner included high amounts of protein but were too low in the energising carbohydrates and healthy fats she needed. The relentless pace of Bridget's life saw her over-training and under-eating, a paradox that left her energy levels erratic and her body in a constant state of injury or illness. She was sacrificing precious sleep to fit in early-morning training sessions, which dropped her energy levels even further.

Her transformation began with a series of strategic interventions aimed at boosting her energy levels and fuelling her body and workouts better. To fuel her training sessions Bridget started eating Medjool dates with a spoonful of peanut butter before her workouts. Then, she ate breakfast within an hour of finishing her workout, to fuel for recovery and her busy workday ahead. Her lunches were revamped to include legumes and whole grains, while sweet potatoes, wholemeal pasta and brown rice became mainstays in her dinners, providing her with sustained energy to power her morning workouts the next day. Healthy fats were also included at each meal for energy, cellular health and hormone function.

Bridget introduced a non-negotiable full day of rest every week, and cut out her second workout on Wednesdays, allowing her body the time it needed to recharge and recover. The benefits of these diet and lifestyle adjustments were undeniable. After adjusting her macronutrient profile to better support her lifestyle, Bridget's body responded by shedding 2.4 kilograms of body fat over 4 months while preserving the majority of her muscle mass. She felt a newfound vigour, not just in her workouts but throughout her workday. By re-engineering her approach to nutrition and training, Bridget had unlocked a consistent stream of energy that propelled her through long corporate hours and tough CrossFit sessions alike. She was no longer just surviving in her demanding world, but now thriving and enjoying a healthier relationship with food that properly supported her goals.

How much carbohydrate do I need?

Traditionally, based on the understanding that muscles are primarily fuelled by carbohydrates, active individuals were recommended to base their diet around carbohydrate-rich foods. It was believed that the more active a person, the greater their need for carbs. However, modern experience has modified this view because the vast majority of people now lead predominantly sedentary lifestyles, as, generally speaking, our incidental exercise has dramatically reduced. While we may be relatively active for some part/s of the day, we also spend many more hours sitting – at a desk, in a car or on public transport, and on the sofa in the evenings. Based on a typical day, our need for carbohydrates has reduced.

The amount of carbs we need largely depends on how much we move, which all up may be less than you think. If you spend all day on your feet and have very little body fat, you will need to ingest more carbohydrates than someone who sits all day, does not work out and has insulin resistance. Similarly, on the days you train for an hour or more at high intensity, you will need more carbs than on a sedentary day when you barely leave the house.

An average adult requires around 30 to 50 per cent of their daily calories to come from carbohydrates. This range accounts for varying size, age and body composition, and also depends on weight, exercise, medical conditions and health goals. Carbohydrate requirements vary significantly between individuals, and are further affected on a daily basis by activity levels.

In simple terms:

- A diet of **50 to 60 per cent carbs** is a typical Western diet that features heavy carb-based meals centred around rice, pasta, grains and cereals, and includes snacks like crackers, fruit and biscuits throughout the day. This relatively high-carb intake means fat stores are unlikely to be burnt unless several hours of physical activity are also happening each day alongside a calorie deficit.

- A diet of **30 to 50 per cent carbs** is moderate – where carbs are smaller side serves rather than the dominant meal base, and calorie requirements are balanced by proteins, fats and insoluble fibre. When followed as a means to achieving an overall calorie deficit, this will generally facilitate 1 to 2 kilograms of fat loss each month.

- A diet of **10 to 30 per cent carbs** is a low-carb or even ketogenic diet in which protein- and fat-rich foods make up most of the caloric intake. Being a focused means to achieve caloric deficit and because fat is burnt preferentially, these diets can be an effective way to drop kilos quickly, but they can be difficult to sustain and even dangerous for some.

If you are unsure of how many carbs you are typically eating, it could be worth downloading a monitoring app to check out your numbers (remembering these are a rough guide only). While we discourage a fulltime focus on calorie counting, using these apps occasionally to check your current intake can be useful. The general guide for a moderate-carb diet is 120 to 200 grams of carbs per day, adjusted for body size and activity.

As clinical dietitians, we know that theory and real life are two different things. When it comes to reviewing eating behaviours, we often find that while people may think they have a low-carb diet, often they're actually eating the wrong balance of carbs. For example, this could be not having enough carbs at breakfast but then overdoing things with heavy rice- or quinoa-focused 'salads' at lunch, or consuming (often uncounted) snacks, coffees and juices throughout the day. The timing and proportion of carbs is just as important as the total amounts – a topic we'll give full focus during the Burn phase, in Chapter 9.

If you're trying to reduce your carb intake it's important to watch the little extras that slip in, which often has to do with portion size or mindless grazing – large, grain-based salads, large slices of Turkish and sourdough breads, rows of rice crackers, juices and milky or sugary coffees. These can add 50 grams or more of carbohydrate to our day without us realising it, explaining why we're not getting the weight-loss results we are looking for.

ISN'T LOW CARB BETTER FOR FAT LOSS?

As carbs are the primary fuel for the muscles, it is a common belief that eating fewer carbs means you will automatically burn a greater amount of fat. This is only partly true. The body prefers to burn carbs in the form of glucose as its primary energy source, so the early stages of a low-carb diet generally deliver impressive results. But if carbs are restricted to a great enough extent for a prolonged period, the body will not only shift to burning fat, but will slow its metabolic rate, too. Once your metabolic rate downshifts, the body ultimately burns fewer calories overall.

This effect can be observed in individuals who lose a lot of weight initially using a low-carb approach but find it difficult to maintain once they return to their usual carbohydrate intake. Being permanently restricted to a true low-carb diet, where carbs are less than 20 per cent of total calories or just 50 to 80 grams per day, can be challenging to stick with long term.

How to best consume carbs

Choose good quality carbs

Not all carbs are equal. They range from 'simple carbohydrates', like the single sugars of glucose and fructose (among others), to 'complex carbohydrates' being combinations of sugars, starches and fibre found in grains such as rice and wheat, which we use to make breads and cereals. Carbs can also be grouped according to their glycaemic index, a measure of how quickly or slowly a carbohydrate releases glucose into the bloodstream. Those that release glucose more slowly into the bloodstream, such as legumes, wholegrain bread and stone fruit, are called low GI foods, whereas foods like processed white bread, certain types of rice and tropical fruits release glucose into the bloodstream relatively quickly, are called high GI foods.

Your energy needs should determine your choice of carbs. Ideally, unless you're about to run a short fast race, it's best to opt for complex carbs and low GI to help smooth out your blood-sugar spikes and deliver sustained energy. Better still, time your eating with movement, and combine carbs with fats and protein or in low/high GI combinations, to reduce their glycaemic load.

Combine carbs with proteins and fats

One of the most controllable factors impacting energy regulation is the macronutrient balance of your meals. Often our meals tend to be carbohydrate heavy, courtesy of large slices of bread and portions of rice, noodles, pasta or potatoes. Snacks often feature milky coffees, fruit, crackers and bars, especially the convenient packaged products that are quick to grab and eat. In turn, these result in the fluctuating blood glucose levels we've discussed.

On the other hand, making a concerted effort to always eat carbohydrate-rich foods with protein, a controlled portion of good fat and ideally a couple of vegetable serves (fibre) will help to slow digestion and keep blood glucose levels more tightly controlled so you are less vulnerable to glucose highs and lows and subsequent cravings.

Move after meals

The more you move, the more blood circulates around the body, facilitating digestion and metabolism. Not only will increased blood flow instantly make you feel more alert, but facilitating digestion will help to reduce feelings of heaviness and discomfort, which can be common after eating – especially if the meal was high in carbs. Moving will also stimulate the muscles to utilise glucose, helping to further regulate glucose levels in the bloodstream. Even if you can only manage to move for a few minutes after eating, it will make a significant difference to your energy levels for the next few hours and burn glucose that might otherwise be stored in your body as fat.

Still feeling fatigued?

If you have managed to put into practice your newfound knowledge around what carbs to eat and when, but still find yourself struggling with your energy levels, it's worth noting that several things can and do affect our 'feel-good' factor. Energy, vitality and fatigue affect both our physical and mental state and concern not only how we physically feel but also our emotions and brain function.[30]

Like many women, you might regularly ask yourself, 'Why am I so *tired*?!' Our modern life likes us to have every hour of the day scheduled and 'hustling hard' is often worn like a badge of honour. Many women are up before the sun to exercise, then work a full day before coming home to social or family commitments, not to mention the often-long commute to work.

If you reach a point of feeling totally exhausted, the simplest answer is to get some rest. Take a week to look after yourself: schedule some naps or longer sleep-ins, reduce the social calendar and drop the exercise. If this helps, it is a good indication that regularly including a little more rest and recovery in your everyday life could be beneficial – as our case study Bridget found. During this period, take some time to reflect on your current lifestyle and see whether you have gradually developed any habits that are contributing to your feelings of fatigue.

Reasons why you may be feeling overly fatigued

You're skipping meals
If you skip meals, you skip regular energy going into your body. Just like a car, your body needs regular 'fuel' to maintain stable energy levels.

You're eating too many high GI or ultra-processed foods
Many busy people grab a quick snack bar, drink or meal replacement on the run, believing that if they're 'meeting their macros' they remain on target. This isn't an issue occasionally, but if it starts to become a regular thing, you will not be doing your energy levels any favours. Fresh is always best and whole foods like fruits, grains, vegetables, legumes and lean proteins offer additional

nutritional benefits over any processed foods. When combined right, they generally help keep your blood sugar levels more stable, which can be helpful from a consistent energy perspective.

Your iron is low

Iron deficiency is the most common nutritional disorder, affecting 20 to 25 per cent of the world's population, and is more likely in women of reproductive age because of menstrual blood loss.[31] Despite this, it is not 'normal' and low iron should be investigated properly by a doctor. If you are going through pregnancy or the postpartum period, or exercise regularly at higher intensities, or have recently given blood or had weight-loss surgery, you may be at risk for lower iron levels. If you're feeling tired and haven't had a blood test for iron in the last 6 to 12 months, it might be worth seeing your doctor.

You're not getting enough nutrient-rich foods

Busy women need several key nutrients to regulate metabolism, hormones and energy levels. Along with iron, it is always worth checking to make sure you are getting enough iodine, zinc, essential fats and chromium. With regards to improving the functions that underpin our body's energy systems, the B vitamins (B1, B2, B3, B5, B6, B8, B9 and B12), vitamin C, iron, magnesium and zinc have recognised roles in these processes.[32] In Chapter 6 we look further at certain nutrient-rich foods that tick the box on these essential micronutrients.

You need to move your body more

It goes without saying that few of us are as active as we need to be. Is it any wonder we feel so tired and lethargic when we spend the majority of the day sitting? Incorporating some vigorous activity into your day, even if it is just 5 to 10 minutes daily, is a crucial step towards optimising your energy levels. This may translate into an interval exercise class at lunchtime, 10 minutes of home gym exercises each morning or utilising a skipping rope each ad break during your favourite TV show. Whatever your choice, moving your body a little more is important if you have a largely sedentary job.

You're overdoing the caffeine

The ironic thing about consuming coffee and other 'energy' drinks to help banish your fatigue is that they are just as likely to leave you feeling even worse than before you consumed them. Though these stimulants give you an initial 'hit' of energy, they also deliver a subsequent 'drop' once the stimulant has been metabolised.

USE CAFFEINE WISELY

While caffeine-rich drinks and supplements are the go-to energy boost of many, they can also be your worst enemy, because while they will give you a hit of energy for 60 to 90 minutes, after the body metabolises the caffeine they are also likely to result in a subsequent energy low. This is not to say that caffeine cannot be used to manage your energy levels, but rather that timing is the key. Ideally, consume caffeine with food, to help buffer its effect, and know your tolerance. For example, a regular coffee contains roughly 100 mg of caffeine, while a large contains double this, and especially large amounts of caffeine will be more likely to result in an energy low.

You're over-exercising

While under-exercise is common, some of us can be found at the other end of the activity spectrum. If you can't remember the last time you had a day off training, find yourself regularly injured or are doing more than one session a day, it might be time to reduce your exercise levels in order for your body to find its energy again.

Your sleep is not optimised

Are you sleeping enough? In its scientific reviews, the Sleep Foundation suggests that adults need at least 7 hours of sleep a night and that women need more sleep than men. They also note that, typically, women's sleep is more disrupted due to various factors including hormones, care-giving, insomnia and anxiety, which reduces overall sleep quality.[33] If you are sleeping enough but your sleep is not optimised, you may have a medical condition like sleep apnoea, or your sleep may be of poor quality due to your sleep environment (for example, your bedroom is too hot or too light) or too much screen time before bed. Some drinks such as alcohol and coffee may also disrupt the quality of your sleep.

Your hormones are disrupted

Our hormones – in particular ghrelin, leptin, cortisol, oestrogen and insulin – can have a significant impact on our energy, as they affect our appetite, metabolism, mood, sleep and stress levels. These are discussed further in Burn. But if you are struggling with these issues and nothing you do seems to help, they may warrant further investigation medically. Women experience significant hormonal shifts throughout the lifespan and getting support from your GP and health practitioners can be invaluable through these transitions.

Nourishing energy

When we recognise the factors that can impact our daily experience of energy, we can see that, generally, we have some control over them. With a few smart choices each day, we can choose to get off the blood sugar rollercoaster, enjoy carbs in more clever ways, and tackle fatigue and hormonal shifts as they arise. Now it's time to dive into another macronutrient: protein, often overlooked by women but an incredible dietary tool, especially as we age.

CHAPTER 5

NOURISH FOR STRENGTH

In the previous chapter we learnt how our bodies convert food to energy, focusing on carbohydrates as a primary source. In this chapter we learn how protein has an equally strong impact on this metabolic process. Protein plays an incredibly powerful role in the function of our bodies, our metabolism and in assisting with weight management. Arguably, for these reasons it becomes even more important as we age. While a much-discussed topic, we find that many of our clients don't fully understand protein's potential to support them on their health and weight-loss journeys.

Consuming the right amount of protein for our body and goals helps keep us fuller for longer, which can reduce snacking and mindless or impulse-driven eating. It supports the development and ongoing health of our muscles, which in turn is beneficial for fat loss. Plus, protein-rich foods tend to tick the box on a lot of other essential nutrients as they often contain zinc, selenium, iron, omega-3 fats and calcium, all of which are really important for maintaining our health more broadly.

Through our practice, we notice that many women aren't consuming enough protein in certain meals, or the right types, and it's a big missed opportunity. Getting good amounts of protein each day is not just for gym bros – it's important for women, too, no matter our age. In fact, lack of protein is often a key contributor to malnutrition in the elderly.

So, this chapter is all about highlighting the why, what and how of protein so it can become a truly powerful part of your nourishment platform. You'll learn how to integrate it seamlessly into your daily food patterns without the need to be chugging protein shakes at every meal!

The power of protein

Protein per gram contains 4 grams of energy, the same as carbohydrate, and is found in largest amounts in animal foods including red meat, chicken, fish and dairy, as well as in smaller amounts in plant foods such as soy, nuts, seeds, legumes and whole grains. Protein, unlike carbohydrate, is not a primary source of food energy. Rather, its primary role is to build skin and hair, repair muscle and provide essential amino acids that are involved in a number of biochemical processes in the body.

Proteins consist of amino acids strung together in complex formations. Of the 20 amino acids there are 9 essential amino acids that the body can't synthesise so these must be consumed in the diet: isoleucine, leucine, lysine, methionine, phenylalanine, threonine, tryptophan and valine (for adults), and histidine (for infants). Protein-rich meals and snacks are also key sources of essential nutrients including iron, zinc, calcium and omega-3 fats.

As discussed in the previous chapter, meals that combine a significant portion of protein-rich foods with fibre-rich carbohydrates will be more slowly digested than meals or snacks that contain solely carbohydrates such as fruit or bread, as the more complex a food, the longer the body takes to break it down.

As a result, these complex foods provide a much slower and longer-lasting source of energy.

A very simple dietary suggestion to help improve the ratios of carbohydrate and protein in your diet, and also help control your appetite, is to try to eat carbohydrate- and protein-rich foods together. Not only will you then have a regular supply of glucose to ward off extreme hunger, but the protein content will help to keep your insulin levels controlled, supporting weight control and metabolic health long term.

Muscle maintenance and performance

The larger your body, the higher your basal metabolic rate (BMR), which, as we learnt in the previous chapter, is your body's energy requirement at rest. In body composition, lean mass (muscle) has more impact on raising your metabolic rate than fat mass – in simple terms, muscles (lean mass) burn more energy. To develop a higher proportion of lean muscle mass, resistance training is of primary importance and protein consumption supports this.

Protein is essential for muscle growth and repair because it supplies the amino acids needed to build and maintain muscle tissue, supports hormonal function related to muscle health, and helps prevent muscle breakdown. In doing this it facilitates recovery from exercise and our adaptation to more demanding exercise.

Metabolism

When we talk about metabolism in terms of protein, we focus on the additional energy requirements it demands. Muscle mass is the type of body tissue that burns calories, so we want to keep as much of it as possible. For this reason, maintaining an optimal protein intake when actively trying to reduce body fat is extremely important if you are chasing body-composition goals.

When our clients say they want to lose weight, what they generally mean is that they want to burn fat; that is, they want to become leaner by reducing body fat and preserving lean muscle mass. Simply 'losing weight' by measure of the scale could mean losing a mix of body fat, muscle mass and water. This is not what most clients want; rather, they simply want to lose body fat and maintain muscle mass to get a lean/toned look. In the case of reducing your calorie intake to support fat loss, keep in mind that if your protein intake is too low, the weight you lose will include a higher proportion of muscle mass, which is not ideal. To counter this, incorporate resistance training as it supports lean muscle. So does eating protein, though to a much lesser extent. To build and retain lean muscle, resistance training is superior.

Satiety

As proteins are not a primary source of energy, they are digested more slowly than carbohydrate and hence play a key role in supporting the feeling of satiety or fullness. Protein helps control blood glucose levels, slows down digestion and, as such, keeps you fuller for longer after eating. Eating more protein can be a good way to reduce your calorie intake as when you don't eat enough protein during the day you can end up feeling more hungry, and thus be more prone to overeating.

Protein and weight loss

If you are trying to lose weight, protein is particularly important for two reasons.

Firstly, when you reduce your overall calorie intake you will also typically reduce your protein intake. If you are eating less than one gram of protein per kilogram of body weight, you may find yourself feeling hungry and lacking in essential nutrients, especially if you are consuming very few calories. Adjusting your macronutrient balance to include more protein can help stave off feelings of hunger as it is the most satiating macronutrient.

The second reason is that consuming adequate protein will also ensure that you preserve as much muscle mass as possible.

A low intake of calories and proteins will naturally lead to some muscle loss. The more we can minimise this with an adequate protein intake, the better it is for your long-term metabolism and weight management. When you're trying to maintain or lose weight, it's incredibly important to preserve your muscle mass, which ultimately helps your metabolism.

Meet Jasmine: eating a poorly balanced plant-based diet

Jasmine came to see a dietitian, determined to refine her plant-based lifestyle. Having just turned 57, she knew she wanted to build some lean muscle, improve her dietary iron stores, boost her energy and stabilise her hormones.

The crux of Jasmine's predicament lay in a persistent hunger, a signal from her body that she was missing the sustenance of adequate protein and fibre. Her iron was quite low, which sapped her vitality, left her feeling perpetually tired and made exercising difficult. What made things harder for her to reach her desired protein intake was that she disliked the taste and texture of traditional vegan proteins like tofu and soy.

Looking at her diet, it became clear that her main meals relied too heavily on carbohydrates (particularly for her age and hormones) and lacked protein. Though she was snacking on vegan protein bars throughout the day, these were all heavily processed and only contained small amounts of protein in relation to her requirements. Her diet also lacked the recommended daily amounts of vegetables and wholegrains.

The turnaround for Jasmine began with the advice to prioritise protein and fibre, two pillars for fullness and regularity. Chickpea pasta became a staple, its fibre-rich content supporting her gut microbiome and its protein curbing her hunger. Quinoa took the place of white rice, a subtle swap with a positive impact on her protein and fibre intake. To boost her nutrient intake she also started using nutritional yeast and lupin flakes regularly in her meals and focused on adding more vegetables and salads to her main meals.

For good sources of plant-based protein she turned to tinned beans and lentils, as well as textured vegetable protein for pasta sauces. Switching from non-fortified almond milk to a calcium-fortified variety was an easy strategic move, and she began adding a scoop of vegan pea protein powder to her morning porridge or cereal.

To support her iron absorption from proteins, Jasmine stopped drinking tea and coffee with her meals (as these can be protein inhibitors) and upped her intake of dark leafy greens, enhanced with a squeeze of lemon juice to better help her absorb the iron. Jasmine snacked on dried apricots and roasted chickpeas, which boosted the fibre, protein and iron in her diet. She also took a high-strength iron supplement as recommended by her doctor.

The benefits of this protein and fibre enrichment in her diet were profound. Jasmine started training at her local gym and saw improvements in muscle mass in just a few months, fuelled by the ample protein now in her diet and the increase in energy levels the extra iron provided. The increase in dietary fibre brought stability to her blood sugar levels, keeping her cravings down, her energy consistent and her digestion ticking along in a positive way. No longer constantly hungry, she enjoyed the peace of feeling satiated after her meals for the first time in years. The increased fibre in her diet set her up for a more diverse gut microbiome heading into the future.

Jasmine's journey to a protein- and fibre-rich vegan lifestyle helped her realise the power of these essential nutrients in her plant-based world.

NOTES FROM THE NUTRITION COUCH
WHAT TO LOOK FOR WHEN SHOPPING FOR BREAD THAT IS MARKETED AS A 'PROTEIN BREAD'

- Check the label: Does it contain significantly higher levels of protein than a loaf of wholegrain bread? If not, you're paying for the marketing and possibly missing out on the nutrients in the wholegrain option.
- As a rule of thumb, a loaf of bread rich in protein will contain upwards of 15 grams of protein per two slices.
- High-protein breads may not be enough to act as the sole source of protein in a meal. If the total protein is not over 20 grams in two slices, consider adding eggs or other protein-rich ingredients to your bread to boost its protein power.

1 October 2023[34]

How much protein do we need?

Now that we know the important role of protein, the next question is: how much of it should we be getting each day?

Unfortunately, it's not as easy as prescribing a certain amount per kilogram of body weight as factors such as gender, activity level and health considerations must be taken into account. Generally, however, research has shown that consuming 1 to 1.5 grams of protein per kilogram of body weight can have benefits for muscle health, especially during weight loss (to reduce the associated loss of muscle) and in older adults.[35]

Can you have too much protein?

Indeed, you can. Protein is still a source of calories, so any additional protein above your requirements is not necessary or advantageous. It is generally accepted that healthy adults do not need more than 2 to 3 grams of protein per kilogram of body weight for any extended period of time, and don't generally need more than 30 to 40 grams of protein at each meal through the day.

And while protein is important, more is not better. Eating protein far above the recommended amounts risks weight gain as you're likely creating a calorie surplus and may also displace other essential nutrients in your diet.

Recently, we heard this story from a new client of ours who, as a female weighing 60 kilograms, should have been consuming around 60 to 80 grams of protein daily, per the standard dietary guidelines. She had recently come off the back of working with a personal trainer, observing, 'I'm definitely stronger, I've put on a lot of muscle mass – but I've also gained weight the whole time I've been following my trainer's meal plan. My clothes don't fit anymore!' It soon became clear why: this client's former trainer had her eating 180 grams of protein a day. To meet those guidelines she was having 3 protein shakes a day and eating minced meat and broccoli for breakfast! This is not the style of eating we advocate – cramming protein in with meals you don't enjoy eating is not a sustainable way to live long term.

Track your protein intake

To find out how much protein you're currently getting, enter one or two days of your eating into a simple tracking app. This can help improve your knowledge around protein-containing foods. You don't have to get obsessive about it – you don't need to count your calories or track your macros every single day – but recording your actual meals and snacks over a standard couple of days might give you an idea of where you're going right or wrong on a day-to-day basis.

Sources of protein

Here are the approximate protein quantities in some common foods, to give you an idea of how much protein they can contribute to your diet.

FOOD	PORTION SIZE	PROTEIN (IN GRAMS)
Beef/pork/lamb	100 grams, raw	30
Chicken/turkey	100 grams, raw	28
Seafood	100 grams, raw	20
Milk (cow's)	250 ml (1 cup)	9
Cheese (cheddar)	20 grams (1 slice)	5
Yoghurt (high-protein)	140 grams (1 pouch)	11
Tuna/salmon	95 grams (1 tin)	20
Egg	56 grams (1 large)	7
Baked beans	250 grams (1 cup)	14
Nuts	15 nuts	5
Protein powder (WPI)	2–3 tablespoons	20

Let's talk about . . . protein powder

While protein powder is not essential to meeting your daily protein requirements, it can be a convenient way to get a concentrated serve of protein in a way that's easy to access and store. For vegetarians and vegans in particular, it can help with meeting protein needs. Choosing the 'right kind' of protein powder can be challenging, however, as there are many different types of protein powder available. Most importantly, choose one with minimal additives and low (or no) added sugars.

The most common dairy-based milk protein is either whey protein concentrate (WPC) or whey protein isolate (WPI), or a mix of both. WPC is about 80 per cent protein by weight, with the remaining 20 per cent consisting of fats and carbohydrates. WPI, on the other hand, undergoes additional processing to remove more fat and carbs, resulting in a powder that is around 90 per cent (or higher) protein. WPI is often favoured for fat loss due to its lower calorie content and higher protein percentage, making it 'leaner'. It's also lower in lactose, which can be better for those with a lactose intolerance or sensitivity.

Vegan protein powders such as pea protein and rice protein are alternatives for those avoiding dairy. If choosing a plant-based protein powder, ensure that the powder has 2.5 to 3 grams of leucine per serving to optimise muscle protein synthesis. Pea protein is a legume-based powder that can stand alone as a complete protein with a good amino acid profile. However, it's typically lower in protein and higher in carbohydrates compared to dairy proteins. Some find its taste and texture less appealing. Rice protein is usually mixed with other plant proteins to form a complete protein source. Vegan proteins often require larger servings compared to dairy protein to provide the same amount of certain amino acids, like leucine, which is crucial for muscle growth.

How do I use protein powder?

Protein powder is a concentrated source of protein and provides the option to get a high quality protein in a small amount of food. A single serve of protein powder is an easy and convenient way to add 20 grams of protein to a meal, and it can be enjoyed in a smoothie, shake or added to snacks or baking to increase your daily protein intake.

Spread your protein across the day

One of the key observations we have with our female clients is that protein is not spread evenly throughout the day and tends to be disproportionate at night. For example, you might get 5 to 10 grams in your breakfast, then another 12 to 15 grams at lunch in a small tin of tuna with a leafy salad, then you're having a big slab of meat or large fillet of salmon at dinner, giving you 50 to

60 grams of protein in the evening (which is far too much in a single meal).

While meeting your daily protein requirement is the primary goal, eating it more evenly throughout the day brings added benefits. As discussed previously, well-spaced and combined eating benefits your metabolic health and blood sugar regulation. Some argue that it also makes it easier for your body to utilise the protein effectively, so if your goal is fat loss or lean body composition – in other words you want to get fitter and more toned – there is some evidence to suggest that spacing your protein across the day can help.[36] As a rough guide, aim to consume a third of your daily requirement (25 to 40 grams) every 3 to 4 hours, across 3 meals per day.

It is very easy to shift your dietary balance to support a slightly higher proportion of protein. In general, all you need to do is make sure that your snacks contain nuts or low-fat dairy, and your meals, a reasonable portion of lean meat, eggs or dairy foods.

Here are some of our top tips for boosting your protein at mealtimes and snack times:

Breakfast
- Use a high-protein yoghurt with your cereal.
- Add a tablespoon of protein powder to overnight oats.
- Enjoy cottage cheese, smoked salmon, baked beans or eggs as toast toppers.
- Swap to protein-based bread/toast.

Lunch
- Add a can of tuna or salmon to your salad.
- Enjoy soup with a slice of protein toast.
- Add beans or legumes to soups or stews.
- Use leftover lean protein from dinner.

Dinner
- Make a piece of lean meat, chicken, salmon or other fish the focus of your meal.
- Add legumes, tofu or tempeh to vegetarian meals.
- Use high-protein pastas or pizza bases.

Snacks
- Include more dairy such as yoghurt or cheese with your snacks.
- Add nuts or seeds to a fruit-based snack.
- Use some protein powder to make energy balls, or add it to a smoothie.
- Look for the growing range of legume-based snacks like roasted chickpeas or fava beans.

THE ROLE OF PROTEIN AS WE AGE

The Australian Government's guidelines suggest that once we reach 70 years of age, our daily protein requirements increase – jumping up to (per kilo of body weight) 65 grams (from 52 grams) for males, and to 46 grams (from 37 grams) for females.[37]

However, global research suggests that these protein recommendations are still too low for optimal muscle function with aging. Furthermore, for retaining muscle during weight loss, research suggests adding a further 1 gram per kilogram for middle-aged and older adults.[38] If malnutrition exists, protein requirements are generally higher, by roughly 1.2 to 1.5 grams per kilogram of body weight.[39]

The power of protein

When it comes to general health, metabolism and weight control, protein is a super nutrient. Not only are protein-rich wholefoods dense in nutrients, but within meals protein also plays a key role in regulating appetite. Consuming adequate protein helps to maintain muscle mass and support the strength of the body. One of the most common issues we see with our clients' diets is not getting enough protein, at the right time, to support their diet- and weight-related goals. For many, a little more focus on this key nutrient is all that is required to take the diet to the next level.

Remember, though, to focus on wholefood sources of protein. Food companies have become very clever at creating ultra-processed 'high protein' foods that masquerade as healthy due to their higher protein content, but whole foods will always be best. This leads us nicely into digestive wellbeing, as a well-fuelled body also needs a happy gut supported by largely wholefood ingredients.

CHAPTER 6

NOURISH FOR OPTIMAL HEALTH

In this final chapter of the Nourish phase, we learn to eat well for optimal health. We learn about the critical role that fats, micronutrients, fibre and fluids play in our diet. Rarely given as much attention as carbs and protein in fad diets, each of them is equally critical to our health and wellbeing, and knowing how to make them work in our favour is often the elusive key to success.

When adjusting the big levers (carbs, protein and movement) has made little impact, focusing on these elements may well deliver the results you've been chasing. For instance, many women suffer from digestive complaints and Leanne's specialist work in the area of gut health has equipped her with over a decade of hands-on experience supporting clients who desperately want to feel better in their digestive systems. In this chapter we'll get to grips with gut health and the interplay between fats, fibre and fluid to help you minimise digestive issues as well as address and manage many common health complaints. We'll also touch on the role of diet as a means to managing good health, such as how certain foods can deliver anti-inflammatory benefits.

In the coming pages we'll see that while often cast as the enemy, fats are in fact necessary for optimal health. We also discover how fibre supports a healthy digestive system, and how fluid is essential in the small matter of keeping us alive. A diet of wholefoods delivers these critical components as well as essential micronutrients, without which we would not survive.

Understanding fats

Fat is a tricky topic in the world of nutrition. On one hand, too much fat, and too much 'bad' fat will result in weight gain, but then we still need *some* fat as the right types play important functional roles in the body.

Fats are the third essential macronutrient. The most calorie-dense macro, they play a vital role in our energy production and storage. They are required for the synthesis of many necessary hormones and to supply our body with essential nutrients for optimal brain function and sustained performance. Far from being 'the devil', we in fact can't live without them – the 'good ones', that is.

Fats form part of every cell in our bodies, and they are especially important for nerve cells, our brains, and the production of many critical hormones. They provide the fat-soluble vitamins A, D, E and K – essential nutrients required by the body that have a range of different functions. The body also uses stored fat as an important source of energy, as per unit it provides more than double the calories found in the same amount of carbohydrate or protein.

There are two main types of fats:

1. **Saturated** fats or 'bad' fats are primarily found in meat, dairy foods, and fried and processed foods. Saturated fat does not have a significant functional role in the body, and excessive consumption is associated with inflammation.[40]

2. **Unsaturated** fats or 'good' fats, which are found in grains, seeds, nuts and plant oils, are more likely to have a functional role in the body, and are less likely to be stored than saturated fat.[41]

As a general rule of thumb, we need only a very small amount of saturated fat in the diet, with most fat coming from unsaturated sources.

Two other types of fats that we hear a lot about and which are especially important to consider are the essential fatty acids (EFAs). EFAs are types of unsaturated fats, commonly known as omega-3 and omega-6. They are essential for healthy development of the brain and eyes as well as forming a structural part of every cell in the body. Despite our often high-fat diets, many people have a low intake of these essential nutrients. The main sources for omega-3 are cold-water fish (such as salmon and sardines), flaxseeds and walnuts; while omega-6 is found in seeds, nuts and their oils.

The main issue with fat intake in Australia is that we get far too much from processed snack foods, fast food, eating out and from fatty cuts of meat and dairy. The mix of primarily saturated fats with processed vegetable oils in these scenarios creates an unfavourable ratio of bad to good fats, ultimately promoting inflammation in the body.[42] Choosing lean meats and reduced-fat dairy and minimising your intake of ultra-processed snack foods will help to reduce your intake of saturated and processed fats, in turn helping to optimise the ratios.

How much fat do you need?

Every person requires a minimum amount of fat, in general no more than 30 per cent of total calorie intake, which translates to just 40 to 80 grams per day for an adult. While there is fat in plenty of foods, we only need a small amount functionally in the diet, and mostly from natural, plant-based sources such as extra-virgin olive oil, nuts, seeds, avocado and oily fish. These fats have a role in keeping the cells healthy, in hormone production and, in the case of the long chain omega-3 fats, in producing a powerful anti-inflammatory effect in the body.[43]

If you are not eating salmon, avocado, nuts and seeds regularly it can be difficult to get this amount, which in turn means you are likely to be having too much saturated fat from dairy and meat. So, if you have not been paying a lot of attention to your fat intake, focus on rebalancing these foods in order to reap the benefits of unsaturated fat, albeit in small amounts depending on your body size and goals.

The average adult female needs 50 to 60 grams of fat each day. While that may sound a lot, if you consider that a single handful of nuts contains 10 to 15 grams of fat, or that a tablespoon of oil is 20 grams, it is easy to meet or exceed these targets, especially if you include a higher fat food within each meal and snack.

Ultimately if your intake of fat is too high, even if it is 'good' fat, you will end up consuming excessive calories and slowing down body-fat loss. So if you eat a 'healthy' diet yet don't know why you are not losing body fat, it may be worth checking if you are consuming too much good fat on a daily basis from the liberal use of oil, avocado and nuts and seeds. This is especially easy to do if you enjoy snacking on protein balls, bliss balls or energy balls, as these often contain nuts, seeds and coconut oil as their main ingredients.

One serve of healthy fats looks like:

1 tablespoon olive oil

1 tablespoon nut butter

30 grams of nuts

A quarter of a large avocado

1 to 2 tablespoons seeds

The key micronutrients

Just as there are macronutrients that combine to fuel the body, a number of essential micronutrients are also required in small amounts to support a wide range of functions. A varied diet will help to ensure that we get enough micronutrients. Of these, there are also some nutrients that busy women need to pay particular attention to, as low levels can have a profound impact on our energy and metabolic function.

Iron

Iron deficiency is extremely common with up to 50 per cent of women at risk of low iron levels, so it is certainly worth seeing your doctor to check that you are getting enough of this important nutrient.[44] Signs of low iron levels include fatigue, breathlessness, reduced immune function, headaches and light-headedness. While you do find iron in a range of different foods including wholegrains and legumes, plant sources of iron are generally not well absorbed.

For this reason, if you are a red meat eater, it is suggested that you consume lean red meat, in small amounts, at least 2 to 3 times each week, to give the body easy access to the iron it needs to help transport oxygen around the body. A small serve of minced meat, a trimmed lamb cutlet, a lean sausage or a couple of meatballs are all good options to increase your iron intake.

It may also be useful to know that when you consume plant sources of iron via wholegrain bread, cereal and legumes, iron absorption can be enhanced when eaten together with foods rich in vitamin C, such as green vegetables, red capsicum and citrus fruit.

Zinc

Closely linked to iron intake, the essential mineral zinc is found in a handful of foods including red meat, shellfish, wholegrains, seeds and legumes, and plays a key role in healthy immune function, new cell development and sexual function. It is estimated that in Australia 1 in 10 women have low levels of zinc, which can impact energy, fertility and our immunity.[45]

As red meat is one of the richest natural sources of zinc, for those who do not include red meat regularly in their diet it is worth paying more attention to including other food sources of this essential nutrient, such as seafood (especially shellfish such as oysters and mussels) and fortified, grain-based breads and cereals.

Calcium

As calcium is found in highest amounts in dairy foods including milk, yoghurt and cheese, a rise in the number of people avoiding dairy, or replacing it with plant-based milks (which are not always fortified with calcium) appears to have had an impact on our calcium intake. With up to half of all Aussie women impacted by osteopenia, (brittle bones), especially as they get older,[46] it is vital to ensure you include at least 2 to 3 serves daily of calcium-rich dairy, or (high-calcium plant-based alternatives such as tofu. And if plant-based milk is your preference, make sure that it is fortified with calcium.

Omega-3 fat

A special fat nutritionally, omega-3 plays a key anti-inflammatory role in the body, and is important for health and disease prevention long term. Despite this, it is estimated that fewer than 20 per cent of Australians get enough of it. While oily fish is one of the richest natural sources of omega-3 fat, other options to add into your diet daily – especially if you have any pro-inflammatory conditions such as PCOS, fatty liver or insulin resistance – include grain-based breads, nuts, seeds and soy beans.[47]

Iodine

The importance of iodine in our diets is rarely mentioned outside of pregnancy, yet it's a micronutrient that is crucial for optimal thyroid function, and as such, one that heavily influences our metabolism. In Australia iodine deficiency is generally prevalent for various reasons, and is a common cause of thyroid health issues.[48] Low iodine levels are also linked to poor brain development in children and impaired cognitive function in adults.[49] With this in mind, if you are not a regular consumer of seafood it may pay to add it to the menu a little more frequently, as seafood – especially shellfish such as prawns, mussels and oysters – offers relatively large amounts of iodine. For non-seafood eaters, choosing an iodised salt is the next best step to ensure you are getting enough iodine in your diet.

The magic of fibre

Although a key component of plants, so technically falling under the macronutrient carbohydrate, fibre is worth considering as a separate nutritional component. Comprising the tougher parts of a plant's dietary materials such as cellulose, lignin and pectin, fibre is resistant to the action of digestive enzymes and, as such, is essential for good gut health and weight loss.

Fibre is key to building a healthier gut. Moving relatively unchanged through our digestive system, it helps to soften stools and increase their bulk, making them easier to pass, hence it's often described as 'roughage' or 'bulk'. It fuels the gut microbiome that supports our immunity, hormones and mental health. Beyond that it can also work wonders in managing our blood glucose and cholesterol and in aiding weight management.[50]

Poor intakes of fibre are something we see often in our clinics as only 15 to 20 per cent of Australians are getting enough dietary fibre.[51] Our convenience culture, and especially the crutch of ultra-processed foods, sees many of us missing out on this amazing nutrient and all the benefits it can unlock. There is also growing evidence that a greater fibre intake is associated with a lower obesity risk in adults.[52]

Fibre is important even if you don't have issues using the bathroom as it helps to feed the beneficial bacteria in our gut. Growing evidence shows that an adequate intake of fibre can reduce your risk of chronic disease, help modulate blood glucose, improve laxation, reduce blood cholesterol[53] and may even help with weight loss and obesity management as diets high in fibre have a lower energy density and may therefore help in moderating obesity.[54]

How much fibre do you need?

In Australia, a healthy adult female should be eating 25 grams of fibre per day and a healthy adult male should be eating 30 grams of fibre per day.[55] However, the latest Australian data surveys show that men only consume on average 24.8 grams of fibre a day and adult women only consume 21.1 grams of fibre a day.[56] The shortfall in fibre intakes is greatest among adolescent populations, young adults, men, those following calorie-restricted diets and those of lower socio-economic status.

Although we encourage most of our readers to increase their fibre intake, it's important to introduce extra fibre into the diet slowly, along with an adequate fluid intake. This allows the gut bacteria to adjust to the change over a few weeks. Increasing fibre too quickly, especially without enough fluids, can lead to negative gut symptoms such as excessive wind, abdominal pain or bloating.

The different types of fibre

Soluble fibre is what we consider the gentle fibre as it dissolves in water to form a soft, gel-like material that can help to slow digestion, keeping you fuller for longer. There are numerous health benefits associated with soluble fibre such as improvements in blood cholesterol and glucose levels.[57]

Insoluble fibre doesn't dissolve in water but acts like a broom and helps to move material through the digestive system and increase the bulk of the stool so it's beneficial for those who struggle with constipation.

Resistant starch is a component of dietary fibre that 'resists' digestion in the small intestine. It passes through to the large intestine where it ferments and can help to feed the good bacteria in the bowel.

TYPE OF FIBRE	FOOD SOURCES
Soluble fibre	Oats, beans, pears, psyllium, apples, citrus, carrots, barley.
Insoluble fibre	Wheat bran, nuts, beans, legumes, wholewheat flour, green beans, cauliflower, potatoes, the skin of fruits and vegetables.
Resistant starch	Under-ripe bananas, cooked and cooled pasta, potato or rice, frozen bread, wholegrain cereals and legumes.

TOP WAYS TO ADD MORE FIBRE TO YOUR DIET

- Leave the skin on your fruits and vegetables where possible.
- Aim for the recommended amounts of fruit (2 serves a day) and vegetables (5+ serves a day).
- Add beans and legumes to salads, stews or mince dishes.
- Add nuts and seeds as toppers to vegetable dishes/salads.
- Cook with wholegrain pasta, wholegrain crackers and wholegrain flour.
- Swap white rice for brown rice, red rice, black rice or quinoa.
- Swap white or wholemeal bread for authentic sourdough, wholegrain or a denser type of bread.
- Eat wholegrain oats with added fruit, nuts and seeds.
- Snack on nuts, roasted chickpeas, edamame beans or popcorn.
- Snack on vegetable sticks and hummus or fruit with nut spread.
- Sprinkle wheat bran or psyllium husk on cereal, muesli or yoghurt.

Meet Whitney: how fibre and fat impact IBS ⌂

At 53, Whitney was looking to shed some excess weight, improve her IBS symptoms and gain a deeper understanding of the foods that truly nourished and suited her body. Her meals tended to be high-fat and low-fibre, which would then lead to an over-indulgence in high-calorie snacks driven by her cravings for carbs and sugar. Saturated and trans fats featured too heavily, and she drank a couple of cold-pressed juices per day as she wasn't a fan of tea, coffee or water.

Whitney's pursuit of weight loss was being thwarted by an excess of calories, and her gut was in disarray, manifesting as alternating constipation and diarrhoea – symptoms of her IBS exacerbated by a diet rich in fats and liquid fruits and low in dietary fibre. Stationary days at a very stressful desk job plus a lack of formal exercise contributed to her symptoms. So, too, did a fundamental gap in her nutritional knowledge: before consulting with her dietitian, she had no idea about the food and lifestyle triggers that would set off her IBS.

The course correction for Whitney focused on achieving a more balanced plate: less fat, particularly from ultra-processed foods, more lean protein, an abundance of veggies (flavoured well so she enjoyed them, not just steamed like how she thought she had to eat them to lose weight) and a modest measure of wholegrain carbs. She brought her cold-pressed juice consumption right down, to once or twice a week, as she realised that the high fructose content was setting off her gut symptoms. Instead she enjoyed sparkling water a few times a day and used cold herbal tea bags to infuse her water. Identifying some other fruits and veggies that triggered her symptoms, she limited them also and focused on adding more pre- and probiotics from foods to assist in fuelling her gut bugs. She found that a probiotic supplement specific for bloating and constipation also helped ease her symptoms.

These changes brought Whitney's gut health into a new era of stability. Her stools became more regular and formed, signalling that her IBS triggers – stress, excessive fat and certain fruits, vegetables and juices – were now understood and managed. Over 12 weeks, she celebrated a 4.8 kilogram weight loss, which brought her BMI into a healthy range and gave her the satisfaction of dropping a clothing size and 6 centimetres off her waist.

Empowered with knowledge and a newfound understanding of the interplay between her diet, symptoms and gut health, Whitney could now dine out and read nutrition labels with confidence. Her body and mind were finally feeling in sync, her gut health restored, and she felt ready to go kick some new lifestyle goals!

Fluid is essential

Fluid is crucial for our body to bring nutrients into our cells, eliminate waste, protect our organs and joints, and help maintain our body temperature. If we're not getting enough fluid, it can lead to dehydration, headaches, poor performance and even impact our digestion and skin.

Humans can last weeks without food, but water is an essential nutrient we can only survive days without. Water is used in our cellular functions, skin, blood, digestion, urine, faeces, perspiration and is even found in our muscles, bones and fat stores. The human body can't store water, so we need to replenish our supplies daily. If you don't drink enough water or fluid, you can quickly become dehydrated, which can be a life-threating condition.

A lot of foods that we eat contain water and this can be included in our daily fluid intake. Our dietary intake alone can make up about 20 per cent of our fluid needs each day. When we eat and digest foods, this process can also produce a small amount of water, roughly 10 per cent of our needs, so we can include this as well. The remaining 70 per cent of the body's fluid needs must come from drinking fluids.

How much water you need depends on many things including your height, weight, gender, activity levels, and lifestyle factors such as breastfeeding or medical conditions. People who need less water are those who lead sedentary lives, live in colder climates or eat a lot of high-water-content foods like soups, fruits and yoghurts. People who need more water are those who are quite active, live in hotter climates, have a higher fibre diet, or who lose fluids (for example, through diarrhoea and vomiting). When increasing your intake of dietary fibre, it is always recommended to increase your intake of fluid because fibre requires water to be properly digested. Soluble fibre dissolves in water.

The average adult needs between 2 and 3 litres of fluid a day (men, as typically larger, fall at the upper end, while women fall at the lower end). Pregnant and breastfeeding women typically need 2.3 to 3 litres a day based on the above lifestyle considerations.

The best way to know if you are drinking enough water is to check the colour of your urine. If your pee is pale yellow or straw-coloured then you are likely drinking enough, but if it is dark brown or orange, you need to hydrate more. Also be aware that it can be dangerous to drink too much water so if you have concerns about your fluid intake, please see a medical professional for individualised advice.

BEWARE HYPONATREMIA

Though it's unlikely for the everyday person, drinking too much fluid can also be life-threatening. Doing so can put the ratio of water and sodium in the blood out of balance, causing an insufficient sodium level, which is known as hyponatremia. Exercise-induced hyponatremia occurs in endurance athletes who over-hydrate without replenishing important electrolytes and has been a cause of death among marathon runners.[58]

The importance of gut health

In recent years, you may have noticed that there is a lot more interest in eating for gut health, with research increasingly showing that the health of our digestive system plays a powerful role in directing our overall health, immune function and even metabolism. It appears that our modern life and the stressors associated with it, along with more highly processed diets, have played havoc with the bacteria naturally found in the digestive system. In addition, our environment, antibiotic use and also chemical residues can disrupt the important balance of bacteria in our tummies. In turn, this means more gut issues, reduced immune function, an increased risk of a number of disease states and even weight gain.[59]

As we learn more about the importance of keeping our gut healthy, the good news is that it is not overly complicated to nourish our gut more effectively on a daily basis. The secrets to success lie in including a variety of plant-based foods in our diet, as well as making sure we are getting the nutrients that are known to build the good bacteria in our digestive system and nourish it the right way.

Go for 30 different plants a week

How many different plant foods would you typically include in your diet each week? Five? Ten? Or do you eat virtually the same thing most days? Of all the scientific evidence available, it appears that a diverse diet full of plants is one of the best things we can do for our gut bugs.[60] Specifically, it has been shown that including at least 30 different plant foods in the diet each week is associated with having a greater range of bacteria in the gut, known to be beneficial for our overall health and immune function.[61] A plant point is awarded every time you consume something with a wholefood source of fibre in it, such as a wholegrain, a vegetable, a fruit, a nut, a seed, a bean or a legume.

Eating the same thing each day might be easy for convenience's sake, but it actually tends to starve your gut bacteria over time. Thirty plants might seem like a lot, but if you make it your goal to always include 4 or 5 plants at most meals, you'll easily achieve the 30 plant points every week. As an example, if you usually have oats with milk, banana and peanut butter for breakfast, change it up every few days to include oats with berries, flaxseeds and milk; or add yoghurt, sunflower seeds, pear and cinnamon. The same principle applies for dinners: too often we see clients eating the standard dinner of chicken breast, sweet potato and broccoli. Although there is nothing wrong with this from a health perspective, you're forgoing the nutrients and fibre your gut could be receiving if you were to sometimes swap the sweet potato for brown rice, quinoa, corn, black beans or even high-fibre pasta. The broccoli is great, too, but we'd also like to see a few other different vegetables on your plate to increase the plant points found in your meals across the week.

Get your probiotics

The human gastrointestinal tract is home to trillions of microorganisms and thousands of different bacteria species, as well as fungi and viruses – collectively known as the gut microbiome. To keep them flourishing, it's helpful to nourish your gut with a diversity of whole foods and also pre- and probiotics.

Known as the 'good bacteria', probiotics are microorganisms naturally found in the human digestive tract that improve the balance of healthy bacteria. Probiotics have been shown to help reduce digestive symptoms such as constipation and bloating by altering the gut microbiota. They also help restore gut flora after consuming a course of antibiotics, which can kill off the good bacteria naturally found in the gut.[62]

Probiotics can be found naturally in some food sources, including fermented dairy like yoghurts and kefir, fermented vegetables like kimchi and sauerkraut, and fermented drinks like kombucha.

Probiotics are also available in supplement form, which can be an effective way to get a daily dose of 'good gut health' for some individuals who struggle to consume food-based sources. However, we recommend talking to your health professional to help find the right supplement for you as there are thousands of probiotic strains available in different combinations and selecting the right mix for your health condition is important. Simply taking an off-the-shelf probiotic may inadvertently cause more harm than good.

Feed the good bacteria with prebiotics

Found in various food ingredients, prebiotics promote the growth and function of different types of good bacteria in the gut. Prebiotics found in various fibrous foods move through the digestive tract undigested and then act to feed the good bacteria, promoting their growth and optimising gut balance. As a result, the gut is healthier and better able to absorb nutrients as they pass through the digestive tract. Eating prebiotics regularly has also been shown to help reduce inflammation in the body.[63]

There are a wide range of foods that naturally contain prebiotics, in particular:

- **Vegetables** such as onions, leeks, garlic, celery, asparagus, tomatoes, jerusalem artichokes.
- **Certain fruit** such as berries, bananas, kiwifruits and apples – particularly if they're organic.
- **Starches** such as wheat bran, soybeans, oats, rye-based breads and legumes.

A lot of food manufacturers are also adding prebiotics to their products and you'll see them show up on nutrition labels in the form of inulin, chicory root, acacia gum, GOS, FOS, psyllium or wheat dextrin. If you have IBS, be careful of including too many of these products as you may find your symptoms worsen the more you have.

If you find you have a sensitive gut, increase prebiotics slowly in the diet as they can cause an osmotic effect in the bowel, which can lead to extra fermentation in the colon, causing gas, bloating, pain, constipation and diarrhoea. Prebiotics are very healthy but sometimes those with sensitive tummies need longer to adapt to them, so start with very small amounts and slowly increase them over time.

Give your gut a break

Just as eating the right foods is important for digestive health, so too is giving the gut a break from eating so the natural microbiome has time to replenish and regenerate. Ideally, we need up to 12 hours each night without food, which is far more than the 8 hours most of us have when we include the late-night snacking. In practical terms this means enjoying your largest meal of the day a little earlier, or pushing back breakfast or your milky coffee an hour or two so you are actually hungry before eating your first meal of the day (not just eating out of routine or habit like the average person does).

NOTES FROM THE NUTRITION COUCH
HOW TO HELP YOUR GUT

- If you experience constipation, focus on increasing fibre slowly and ensure adequate hydration to accompany the increased fibre intake.
- Get moving – even just taking short walks, which can help stimulate bowel movements.
- Be careful of processed high-fibre foods that may contain prebiotic fibres like inulin, which can worsen gas and bloating in sensitive individuals.
- Incorporate whole foods, particularly whole grains and legumes, into your diet to improve stool consistency and regularity.

- Eat regular meals instead of constantly snacking to allow the gut to rest and digest properly.
- For bloating and gas, addressing constipation can often alleviate these symptoms as well. If it doesn't, it might be time to book a consult with an experienced gut health dietitian.

9 August 2023 [64]

An anti-inflammatory approach to nutrition

Inflammation is a broad term but generally refers to a natural response by our bodies that occurs when there is injury or damage to the body's cells. Inflammation can be somewhat healthy and normal and experienced regularly as a result of general immune responses, such as repairing cells after exercise, but can also be chronic or systemic due to disease states such as insulin resistance and autoimmune conditions. This is what we want to avoid, or at least assist in managing comfortably.

Anti-inflammatory eating is a simple yet powerful tool we can use to keep our body healthy, reduce our risk of chronic diseases long term and ensure we live with longevity in mind. Conditions like PCOS, type 2 diabetes, insulin resistance, fatty liver, joint pain, high blood pressure and high cholesterol, coeliac disease and inflammatory bowel disease are all associated with an increased amount of inflammation in the body. [65]

There is no argument that there is often a genetic predisposition for many of these conditions; however, the rapid increase in their prevalence does suggest that our lifestyles habits are to blame as well. The good news is, however, if we can change our nutrition and lifestyle, we can often reduce the inflammation in our body and our risk of developing some diseases longer term. [66]

While there are different approaches to anti-inflammatory diet protocols, from those who advocate avoiding certain foods like gluten or alcohol entirely to others who support a Mediterranean or low-carb diet, there are common recommendations across the range that are useful to follow for good health. Below is a summary of several things we can do to help reduce the level of chronic inflammation in our body.

NUTRITION TIPS	LIFESTYLE TIPS
Focus on the right mix of fat Reduce saturated and trans fats generally found in processed cakes, biscuits, pastry, etc. and increase your intake of omega-3, omega-6 and monounsaturated plant fats, found in such foods as oily fish, extra-virgin olive oil, walnuts and chia, flax and hemp seeds.[67]	**Watch your weight** Overweight and obese individuals tend to have higher levels of C-reactive protein (CRP), which is a marker for inflammation. Studies show when excess weight is lost, CRP generally goes down, too.[68]
Load up on fruits and vegetables The brighter the colour of the fresh fruit or vegetable, the higher the antioxidant content, and the more antioxidants we consume naturally as part of our daily diet, the better it is for reducing CRP and inflammation long term.[69]	**Move your body regularly** Engaging in regular exercise is not only beneficial for losing weight, but it can also assist in lowering CRP levels long term. Aim to do at least 30 minutes of continuous activity most days of the week.[70]
Go green & plant based Studies show lower levels of inflammation when we eat more magnesium from foods such as green vegetables, nuts and legumes.[71]	**Manage stress** Engage in regular stress-reducing activities as the higher your stress, the higher your inflammation may be over time. When you are more stressed, you also tend to reach for more ultra-processed food, sugar and alcohol, which in excess can also increase inflammation over the long term.[72]

NUTRITION TIPS	LIFESTYLE TIPS
Reduce refined carbs Of all the evidence out there about carbohydrate intake, the primary finding is a link between the glycaemic load (GI) of the diet and chronic inflammatory conditions including type 2 diabetes and heart disease. Aim to make your carb choices smart ones with a lower GI rating.[73]	**Cease smoking** Studies show smoking may increase inflammation, so if you smoke, it's time to ditch the habit for good.[74]
Sip on tea Drinking tea (both black and green) has been linked to reduced inflammatory markers in several studies. Just be careful how much milk/sugar/syrup you add; plain tea is best for inflammation.[75]	**Supplements** Good quality nutrition is always best but there is research to support some supplements that may be helpful to reduce inflammation. Speak with your health professional for a recommended dose.[76]

Nourish for life

Congratulations on completing the Nourish phase. Now you are well armed to make smart nutrition choices to build an optimal nutrition platform personalised to your own needs, body and lifestyle. In Nourish we learnt how to eat well for sustained energy, for power and strength, and for optimal health. With this healthy base now firmly established, it's time to look closely at how we can fine-tune our approach to achieve our weight-loss goals.

PART 3

BURN

WHY DO WE NEED TO BURN?

If you have the explicit goal of sustainable fat loss you are in the right place. The Burn section of *Reset, Nourish, Burn* is dedicated entirely to the science of fat loss, and specifically achieving fat loss by utilising strategies that can be easily incorporated and maintained in your day-to-day life.

Weight control is tricky in modern life and many of us experience gradual weight gain over a number of years. We have easy access to high-calorie foods and many of us spend much of the day sitting, which gradually tips the scales out of our favour. While subtle, this simple energy imbalance can leave us vulnerable to gradually gaining weight over time and to carrying extra kilos we would prefer not to have.

As we hope we made clear in the Reset phase, we are by no means diet or weight obsessed and have spent our careers working to change the toxic diet culture. We embrace people of all shapes and sizes and respect that every person has the right to be comfortable in their own body. However, in our daily work and the podcast, most of our clients and listeners are women who feel unhappy in their bodies and have come to us for support. They have reached a point where they feel they have lost control over their weight. They want to know how to safely lose weight and keep it off long term.

In Reset we built the first phase of your sustainable weight-management platform, by changing your diet mindset. Then in Nourish you learnt nutrition fundamentals, and armed yourself with all the knowledge you need to take control of your own health journey. Now with Burn you will learn how to lose weight safely and sustainably, so you can feel in control and confident with your body again, at a weight that feels right for you.

SIGNS IT MAY BENEFIT YOU TO SUSTAINABLY BURN FAT

- Your weight continues to increase gradually.
- You feel you have lost control of managing your weight.
- You are more than 10 kilograms above a healthy weight for your body.
- You are constantly on a diet due to being overweight, yet never get results.
- Your waist measurement is greater than 80 centimetres and increasing.
- Your health-care professional has said you need to reduce weight for your health/lifestyle.

The power of the Burn phase

While there are plenty of quick-fix diet solutions out there that encourage periods of extremely low-calorie eating, or that eliminate significant amounts of carbohydrate from the diet, or that suggest you replace most of your solid food with juices, ultimately, they rarely work long term. In our experience, when it comes to diet and nutrition, if it sounds too good to be true it usually is. The reality is, any diet works – until it doesn't. So if that particular diet or lifestyle plan is not something you can see yourself doing for the long term, chances are you'll fall off the bandwagon at some point, and the weight will all come back on again.

When they're in the dieting mindset, most people assume that fat loss requires constant calorie counting, super strict meal plans and cutting out all of their favourite foods, fuelling the belief that a 'diet' for fat loss is something you do for a short period of time before you return to your usual routine. This is not what Burn is about.

Rather, our approach is based on the notion that we want to develop sustainable lifestyle changes that can be maintained forever. No more going on and off a program. No more restrictive meal plans that do not include your favourite foods. And certainly, no more calorie counting or macro tracking in an app for the rest of your life.

For us, it is about matching the goals you have for your body with a style of eating and way of exercising that fits for you. Sure, we need to create a calorie deficit to support weight loss, but ultimately we want you to think of this new, balanced, nutrient-rich style of eating as what you now do, permanently, to fuel and nourish your best self. Here in Burn, you will learn how to create this life plan for yourself and sustain it. No more quick fixes or extreme fad diets, but rather, consistent eating habits that help your body to be at its best long into the future.

We're excited to introduce you to 4 final principles that will help you burn unwanted fat and keep it off:

1. Find your hunger
2. Time your meals
3. Volume-eat your veg
4. Follow our fat-loss formula

The first 3 are rules of thumb that are easy to remember and straightforward to put into practice within a busy and demanding lifestyle. The last is the meal-building formula that we have developed to help you fill your plate at mealtimes in a way that's going to help you achieve your fat-loss goals while also giving you the nutrients you need. No deprivation – just a simple set of ratios you can use every day.

We share these principles with our clients to support them on their fat-loss journeys and the results can be remarkable. So now you've Reset your relationship to food and learnt more about how to Nourish your body better, it's time to Burn!

CHAPTER 7

FIND YOUR HUNGER

When was the last time you felt really, truly hungry? Although hunger is the physiological sign that it's time to eat, it's not always the key driver behind our eating behaviours. Rather, we tend to eat when it is a mealtime, or when other people are eating, or because we are afraid of getting hungry, or simply because there is tasty food on offer. In fact, the most significant predictor of discretionary food intake is availability.[77] Basically, if food is within easy reach, we will eat it.

The issue with eating when we are not truly hungry is that we tend to lose track of our natural hunger and fullness signals, which means we are often eating on autocue rather than being in touch with our natural appetite. Ultimately, this can lead to overeating on a daily basis – and those small extra amounts can add up over time.

Becoming aware of your natural hunger is a powerful tool to guide food intake, support fat burning and aid in reach and maintain your goal weight. So let's become reacquainted with hunger and learn how to build a habit of mindful food consumption.

Meet Chloe: getting over the fear of hunger 🧳

Chloe, a 48-year-old executive assistant, was very familiar with the highs and lows of yo-yo dieting. Weighed down by the stress of her job, she felt desperate to shed 10 kilograms, break the cycle of temporary fixes and cultivate a lasting, healthy relationship with food.

Chloe's diet was light on protein and heavy on carbs, with snacking bridging the gap between her large-portioned meals, and being vegetarian, she lacked some essential nutrients. Her routine breakfast was a sachet of porridge with fat-reduced milk and she'd usually buy a grab-and-go lunch, often avocado sushi, a falafel wrap or a cheese-and-tomato toastie. She didn't drink alcohol or coffee, but her challenges lay elsewhere.

It quickly became clear in Chloe's first session with her dietitian that she was out of touch with her body's hunger signals, eating as if on autopilot, with snacks stashed in her car, handbag and desk – always within arm's reach. She'd hastily consume meals at her work desk, her focus on the screen in front of her. The fear of hunger haunted her, a ghost from past diets that had left her feeling deprived. Chloe's all-or-nothing mindset towards nutrition had become a real barrier, and she was also burdened by her poor metabolism, low muscle mass, limited protein intake and sedentary lifestyle.

The path to change began with lessons in mindful eating with her dietitian. Chloe learnt to tune in to her hunger, rating it before, during and after meals. She began a food, mood and hunger diary to help her with daily reflection, and that helped reveal patterns and guide her towards balance. She tackled her perfectionist tendencies and negative self-talk, learning to be kinder to herself.

She removed snacks from her immediate reach, reserving just a couple in her car or handbag for true hunger emergencies. With help she was able to reinvent her meals and put much more emphasis on protein, fibre and vegetables, adopting a volume-based approach that allowed her to eat more for fewer calories, while still feeling satisfied and nourished – especially at lunchtime.

Within just 12 weeks, Chloe bid farewell to 8.3 kilograms and instead of seeing the scales as a source of fear, became able to use them constructively as a tool on her health journey. Clothes she hadn't worn in years now fitted, her cravings were massively decreased by her protein-rich, fibrous diet, and she began waking up feeling hungry in the mornings – a sensation she welcomed. Snacks in the car became a thing of the past as she learnt to wait for balanced meals at home.

Her relationship with food was now free from the shackles of black-and-white thinking and she had far more energy each day with key nutrients like iron boosted in her diet. She even found joy in walking a few days a week with a friend, a gentle reintroduction to exercise. Ultimately, Chloe's journey was not just about weight loss; it was about rekindling a positive dialogue with her body and her plate, and she felt totally transformed.

Fear of being hungry

Like Chloe, many people fear being hungry, particularly those with a history of dieting. This fear usually stems from restrictive, low-calorie diets where the hunger is constant as there is never enough fuel during the day. We frequently 'fall off the wagon' with these restrictive diets as the constant hunger gnaws away at us and, eventually, our willpower diminishes.

As a society, we are often taught that hunger is a bad thing, but in reality, hunger is just a signal from our body that it has used up all its fuel and it's time to refuel again. Hunger is just a feeling, an uncomfortable one for most, but one that we ideally learn to sit with, knowing that there are no real side effects from feeling a little hungry at times; in fact, it is completely normal.

More of an issue for many of us is the fact that we have trained ourselves to overeat, often not recognising that we have had enough food until we have overeaten and reached the point of feeling stuffed and overfull. Getting in closer touch with our hunger over time will help us to be able to identify the cues that we have had enough, but not overeaten.

The goal with weight loss is not to constantly feel hungry but instead to feel hungry leading up to mealtimes, which shows that the body has taken the food we've eaten and utilised it for energy. In general, most of us are eating too much, fearing hunger and never giving our body the opportunity to use up all its fuel sources. So, while feeling constantly hungry all day long is not healthy or positive, feeling hungry regularly throughout the day leading up to mealtimes is healthy and even encouraged.

The different types of hunger

Have you ever finished a meal, felt full, then found yourself wandering back into the kitchen soon after? This is something many people experience and something we call non-hungry eating or head hunger – what researchers call 'interoceptive' hunger signals: internal cues for hunger that are not 'innate' but have been learnt or taught.[78]

In other words, your body might 'feel hungry' but it doesn't actually need food. This is distinct from what we term physical or physiological hunger, where your body genuinely requires food and nourishment to continue functioning. Often, these two hungers can be difficult to distinguish as they both feel like your body needs to eat.

Understanding the different types of hunger and how to recognise them in your day-to-day life can be a huge step forward in your journey towards long-term health.

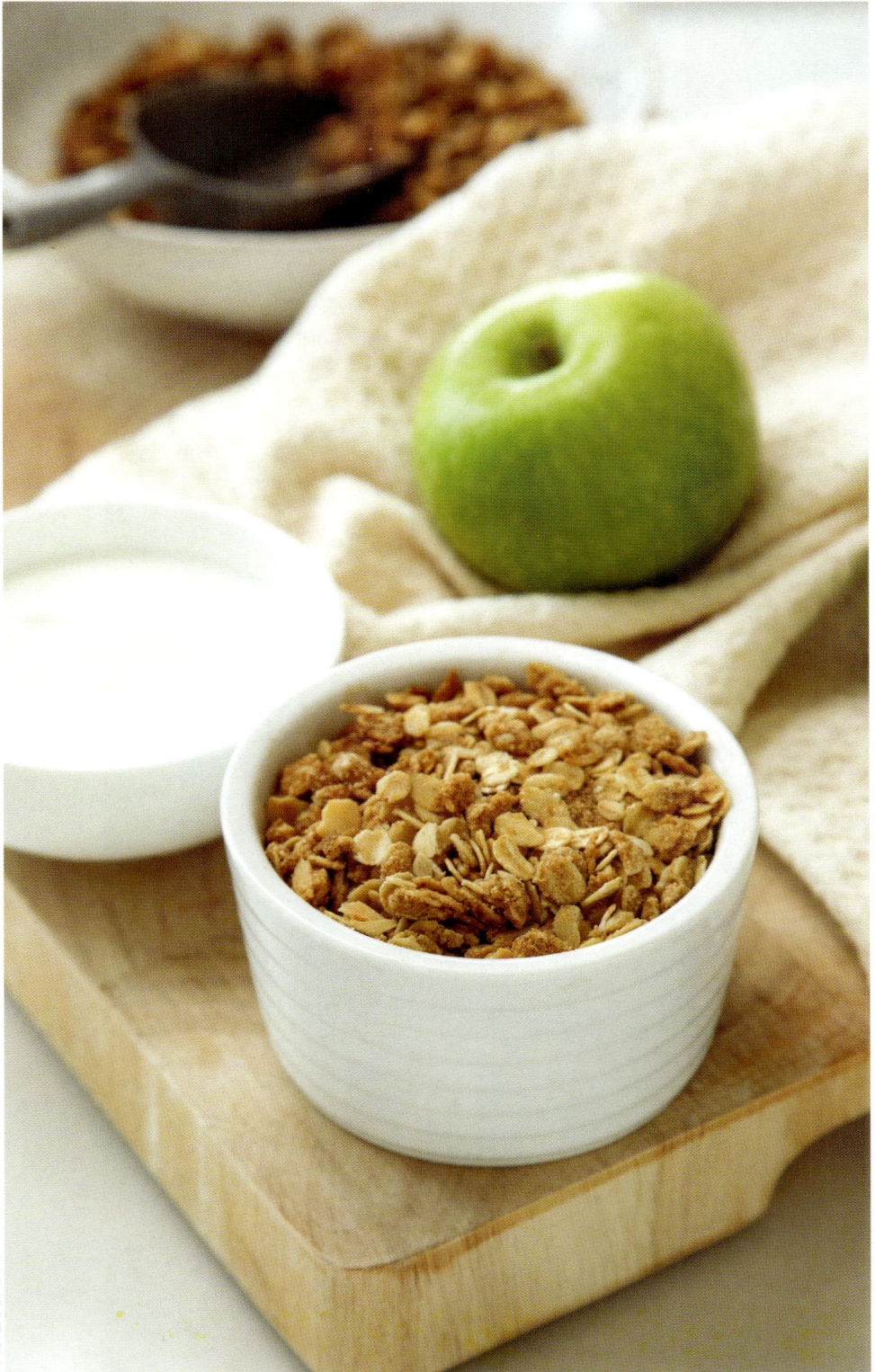

Apple Crumble Bowls, page 225

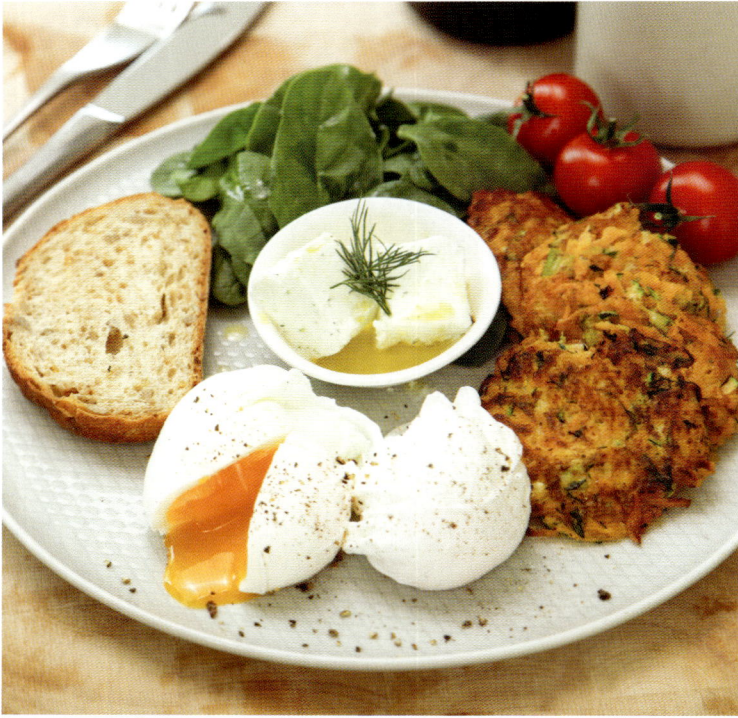

Vegetable Hash Brown with Eggs, page 226

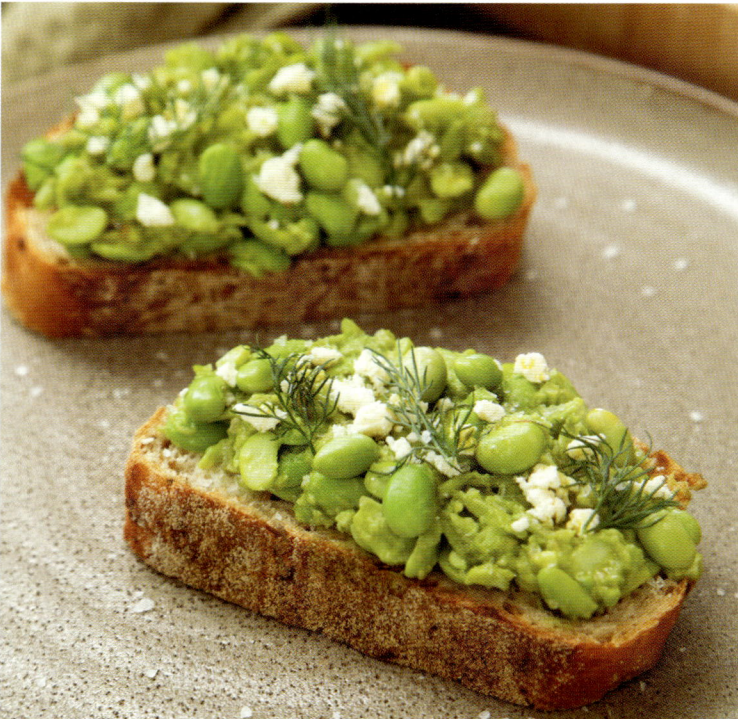

Higher Protein Avo Smash, page 227

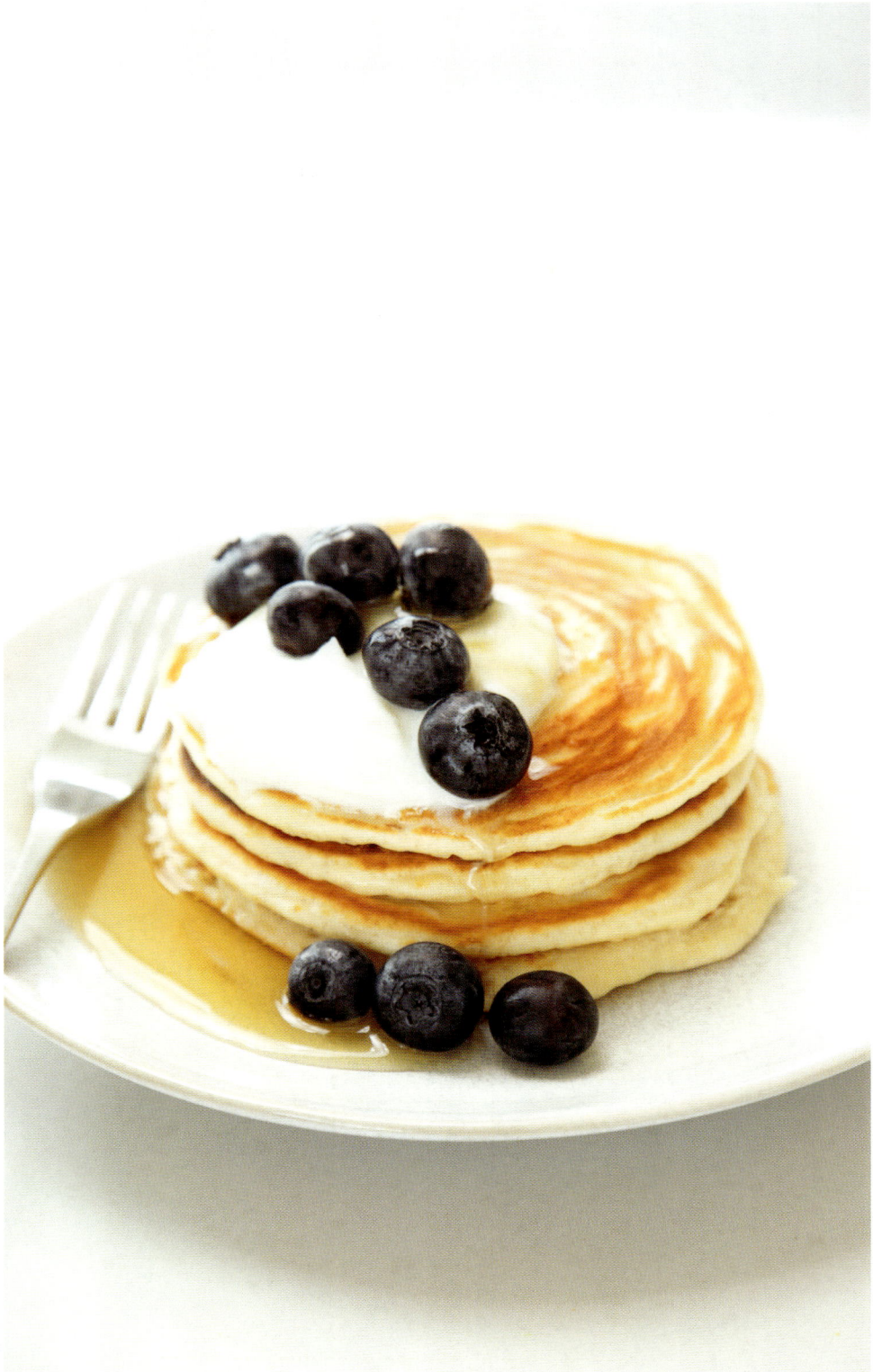

Protein Berry Pancakes, page 228

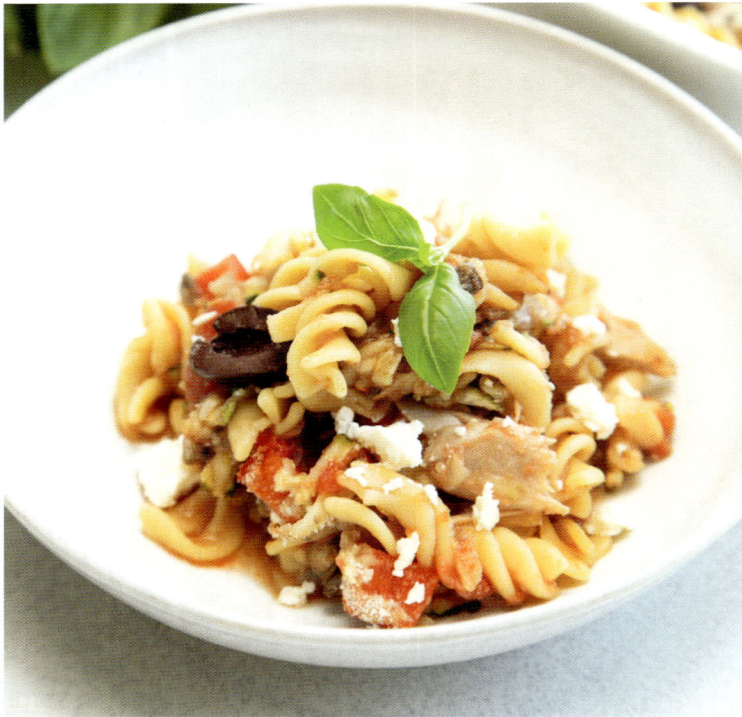

Mediterranean Tuna Pasta Bake, page 229

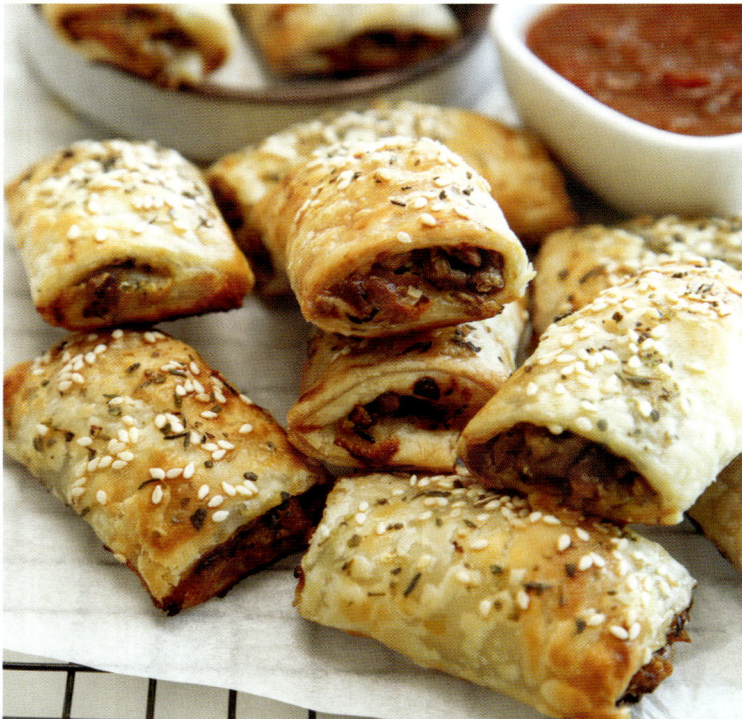

Veggie-packed Sausage Rolls, page 230

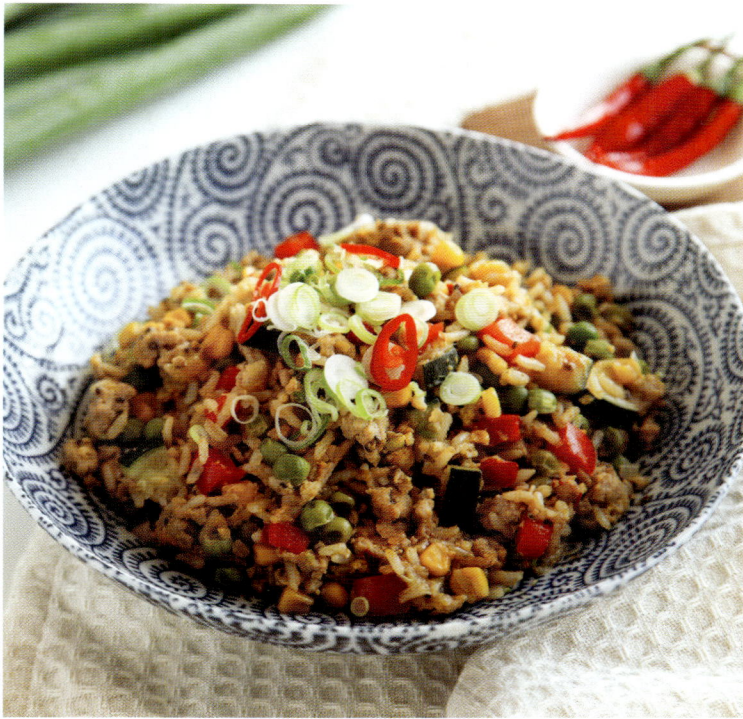

Quick and Healthy Fried Rice, page 232

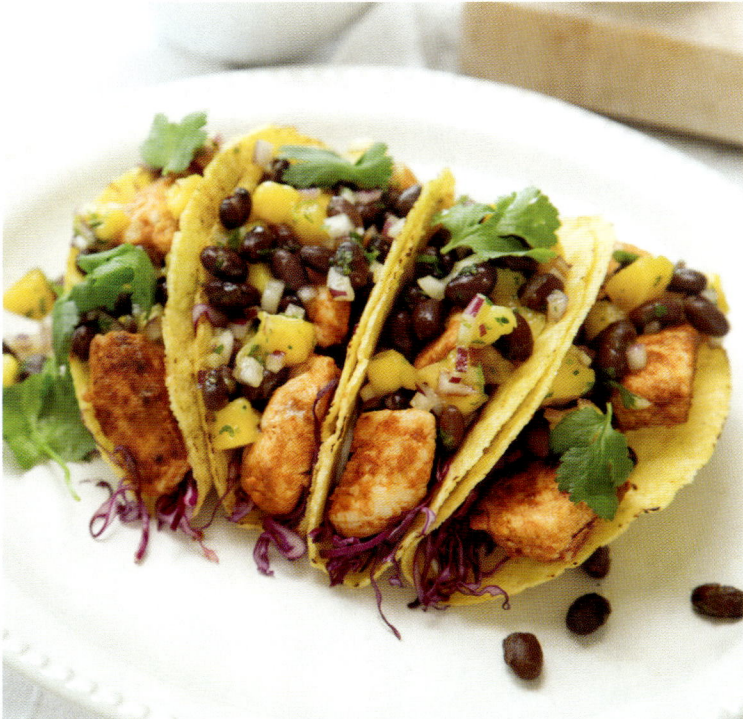

Zesty Chicken Tacos, page 233

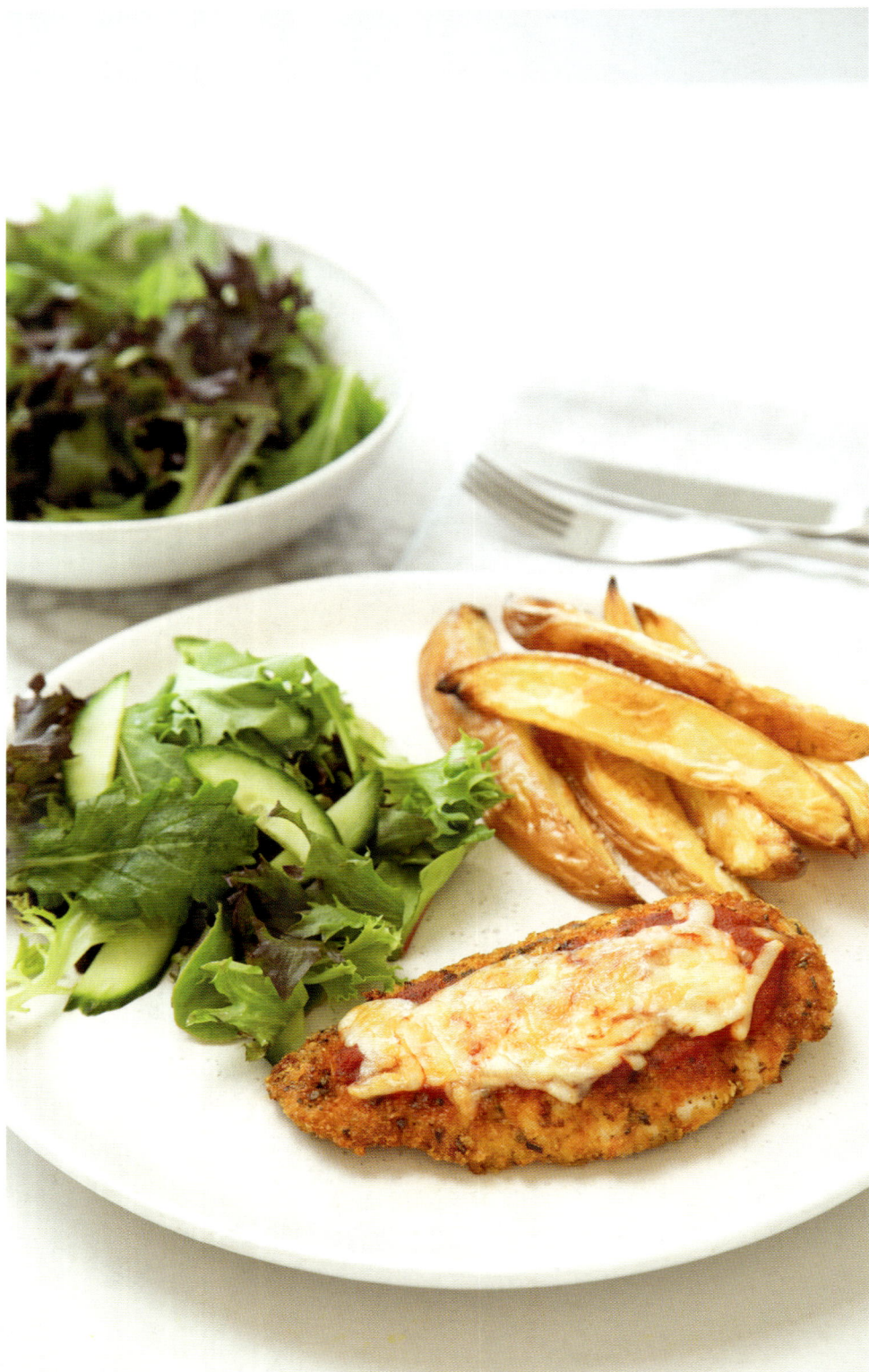

Chicken Parmi, Chips and Salad, page 234

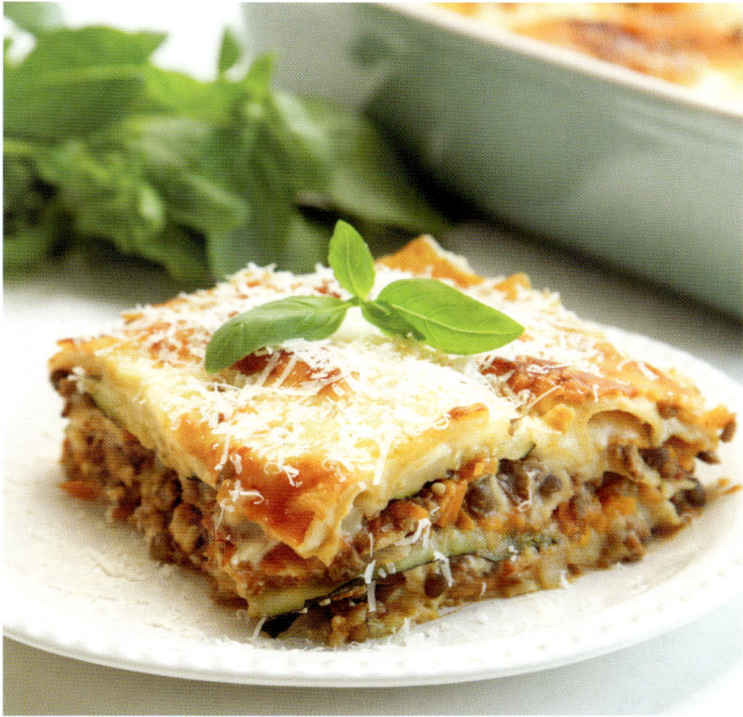

Nourishing Beef and Veggie Lasagne, page 236

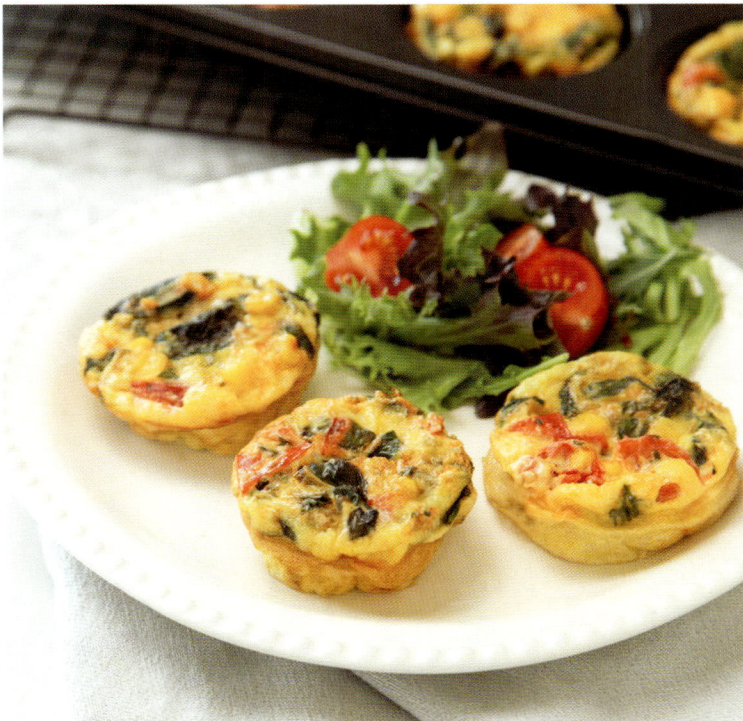

Vegetable Egg Bites, page 238

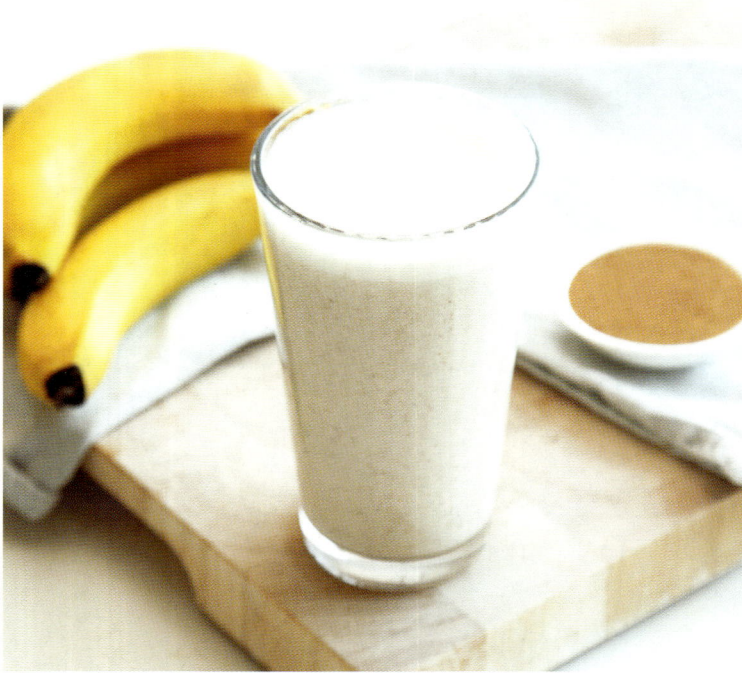
Banana and Almond Protein Smoothie, page 239

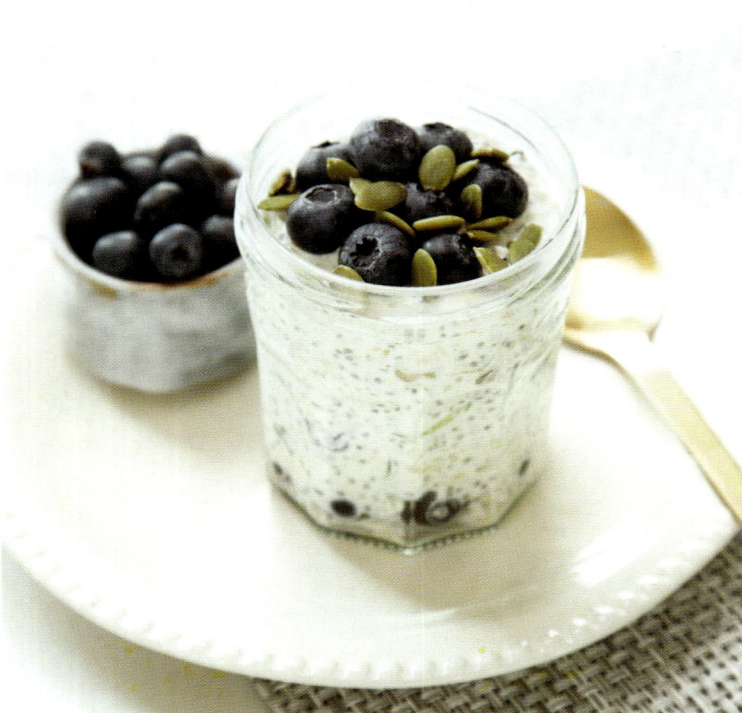
Overnight Berry Bircher, page 240

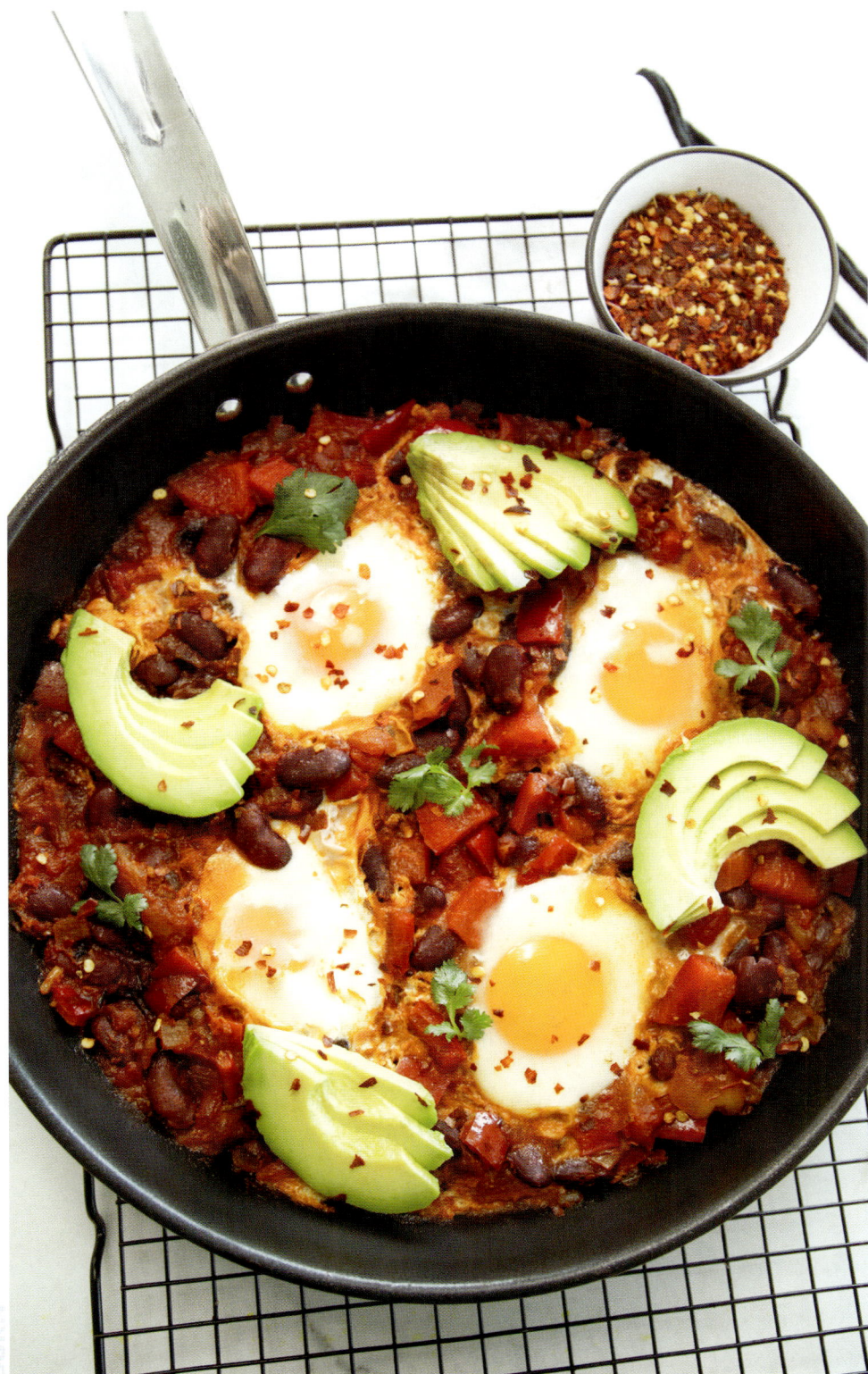

Mexican Eggs with Beans, page 241

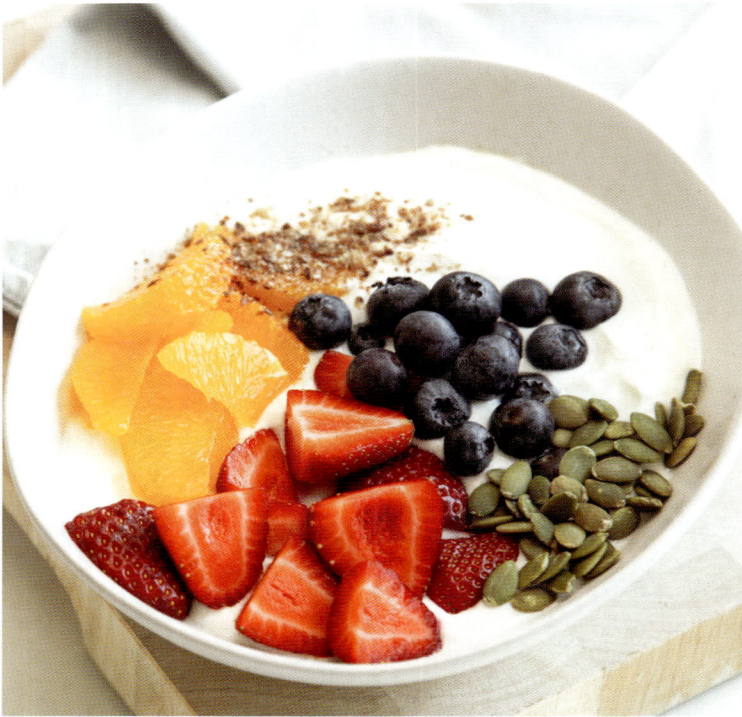

Breakfast Nourish Bowl, page 242

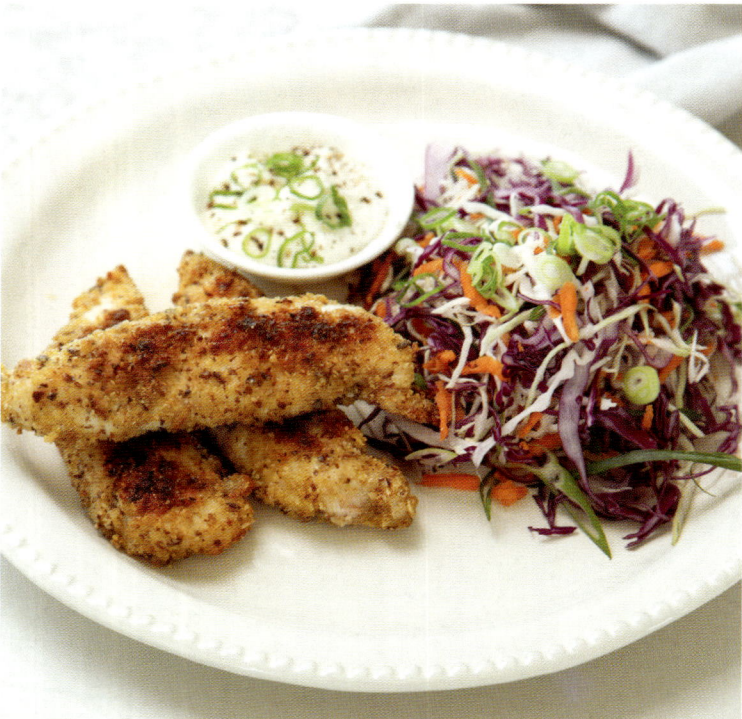

Chicken Tenders with Slaw, page 243

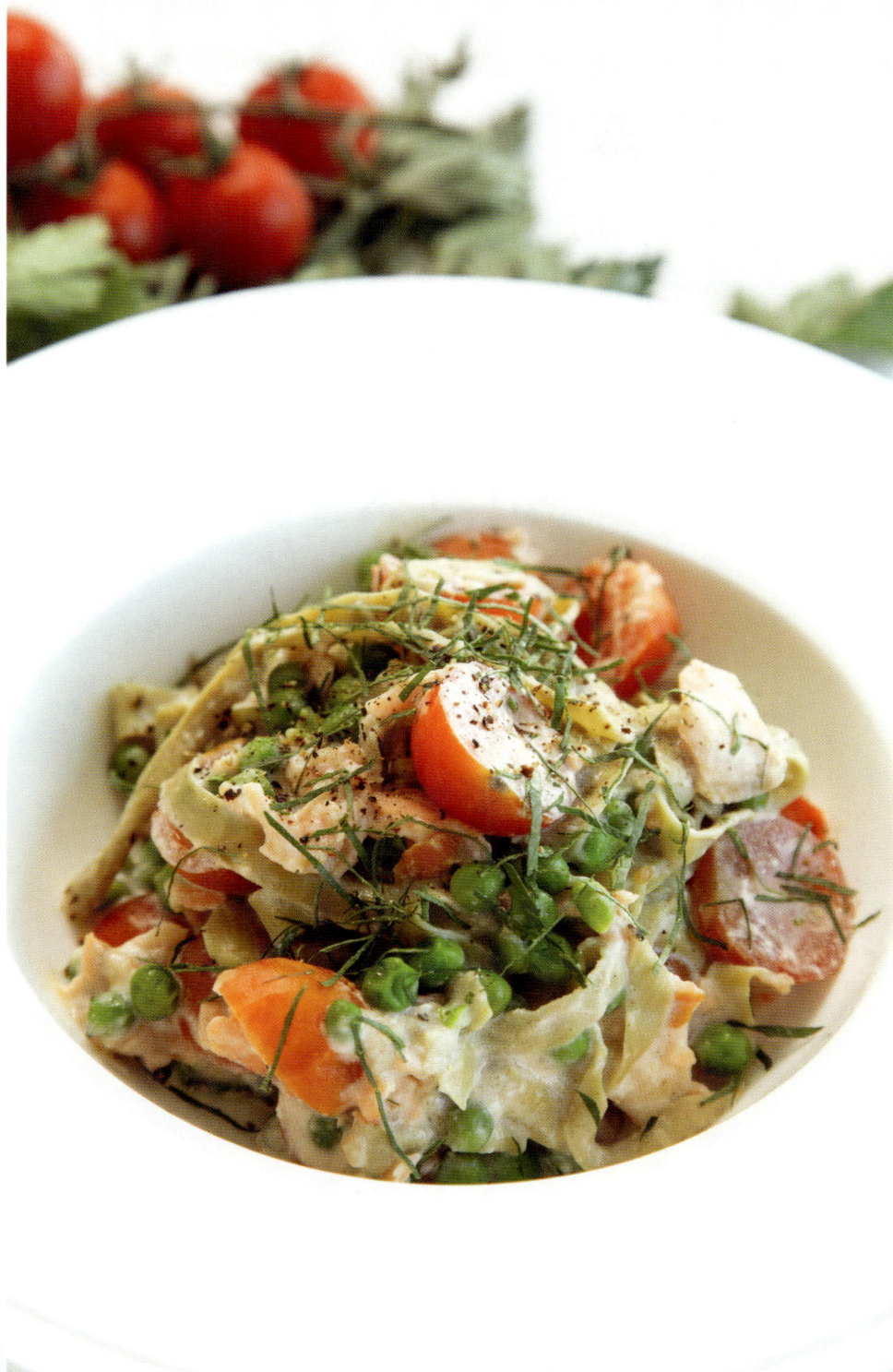

Smoked Salmon and Ricotta Edamame Pasta, page 244

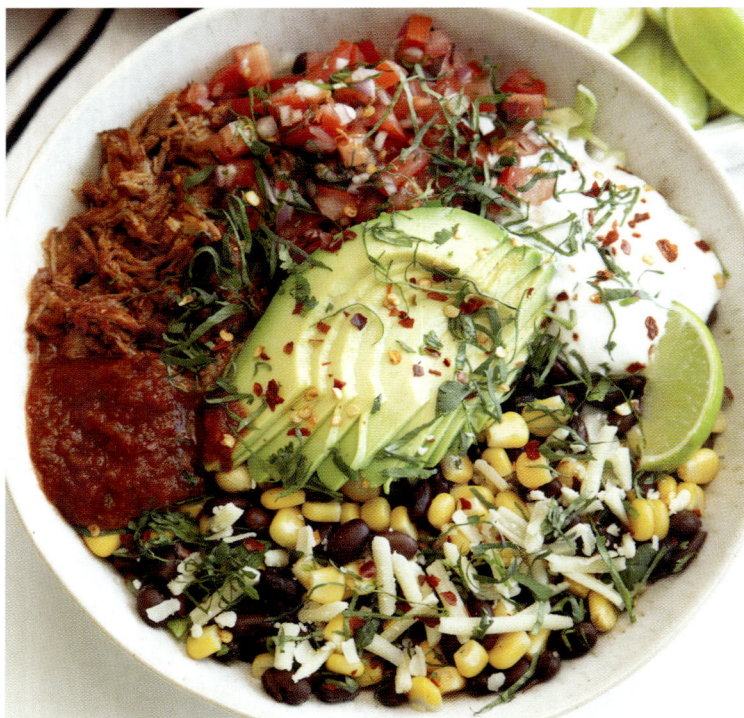

Pulled Pork Mexican Bowl, page 245

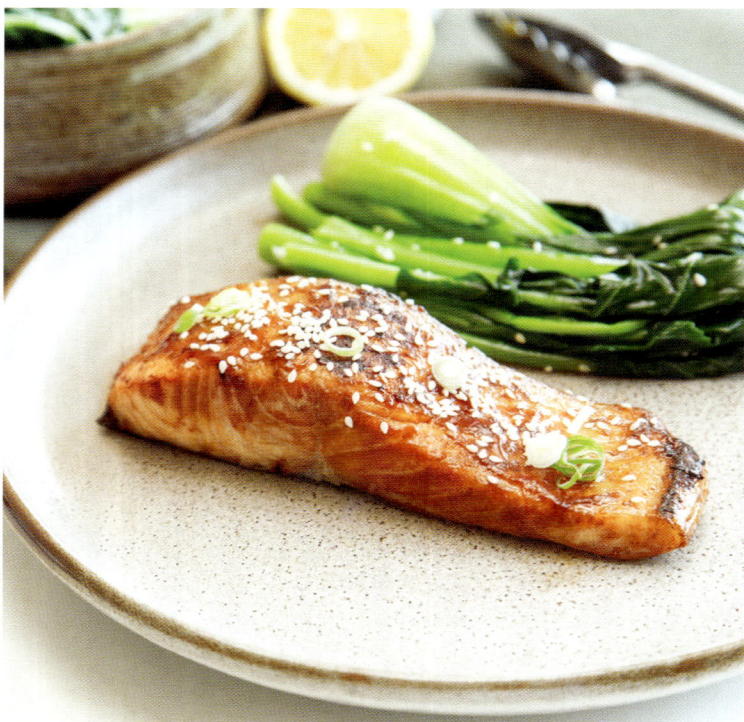

Teriyaki Salmon with Asian Greens, page 246

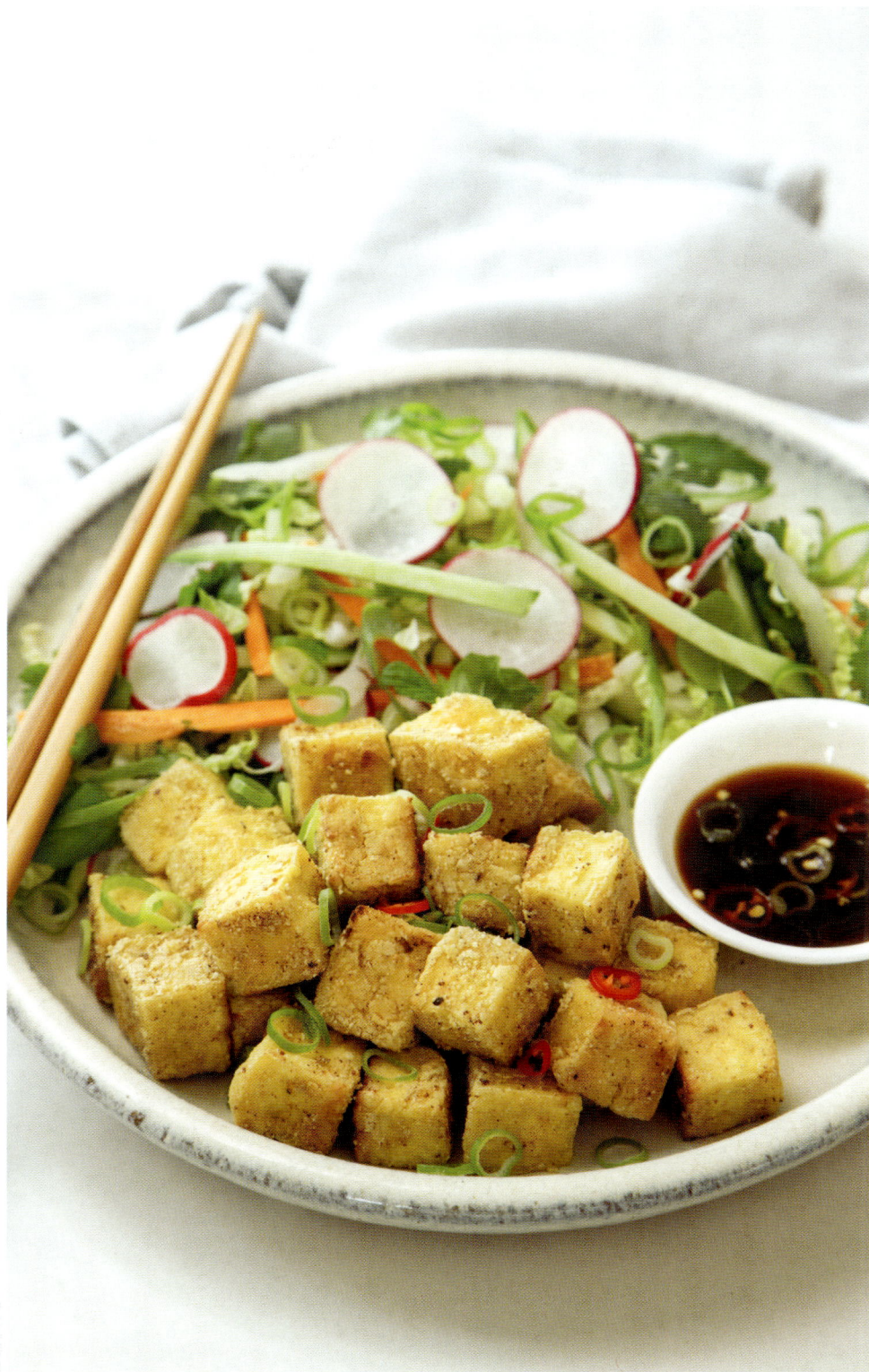

Salt and Pepper Tofu with Wombok Salad, page 247

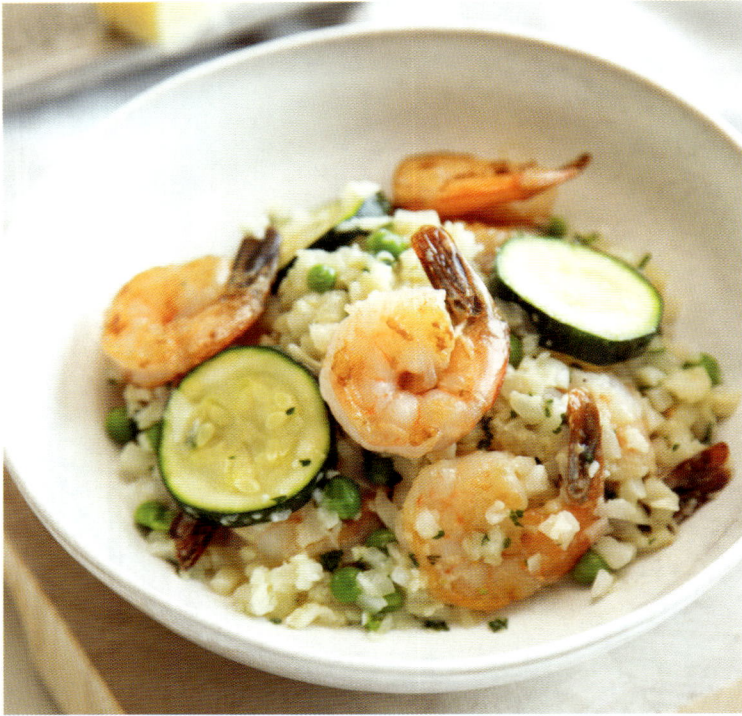

Garlic Prawn Cauli Risotto, page 249

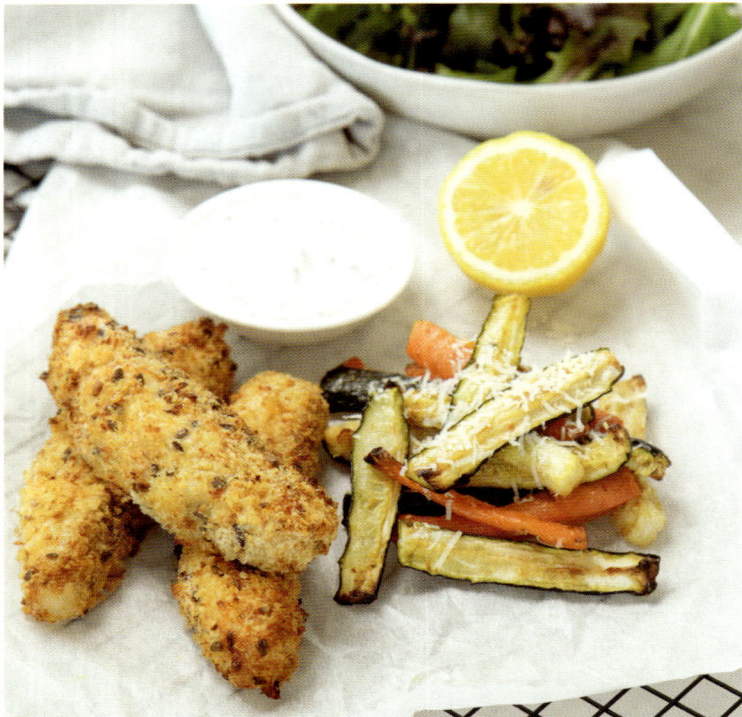

Crumbed Fish Bites and Veggie Chips, page 251

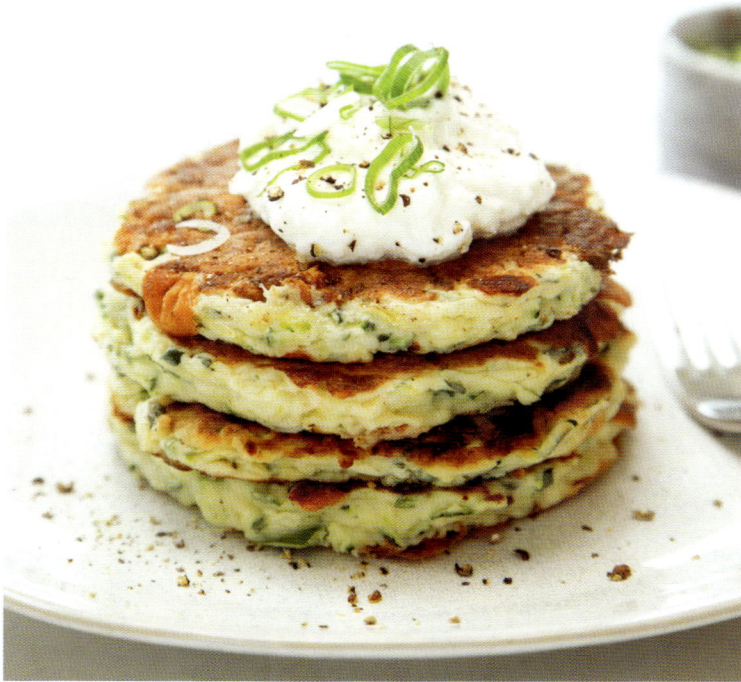

Zucchini and Ricotta Fritters, page 253

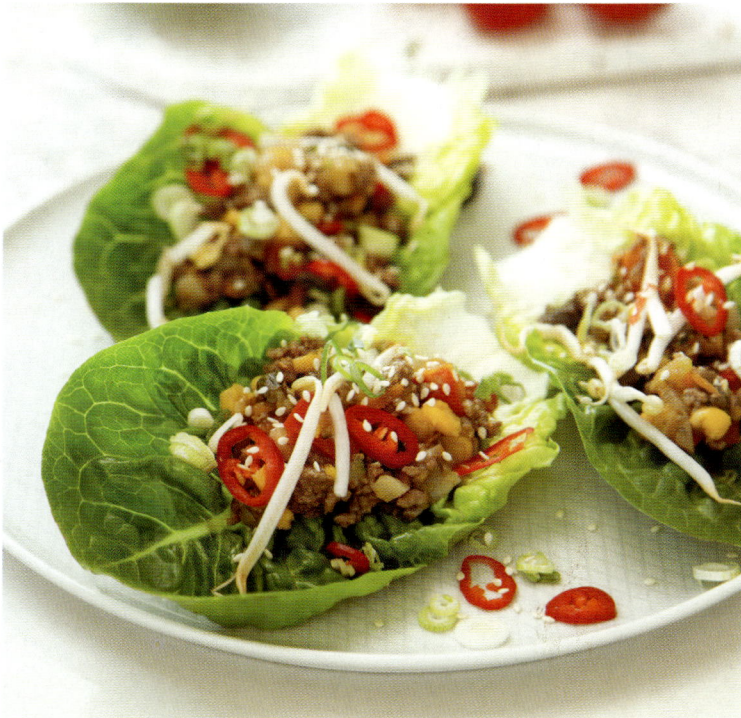

Beef San Choy Bow, page 254

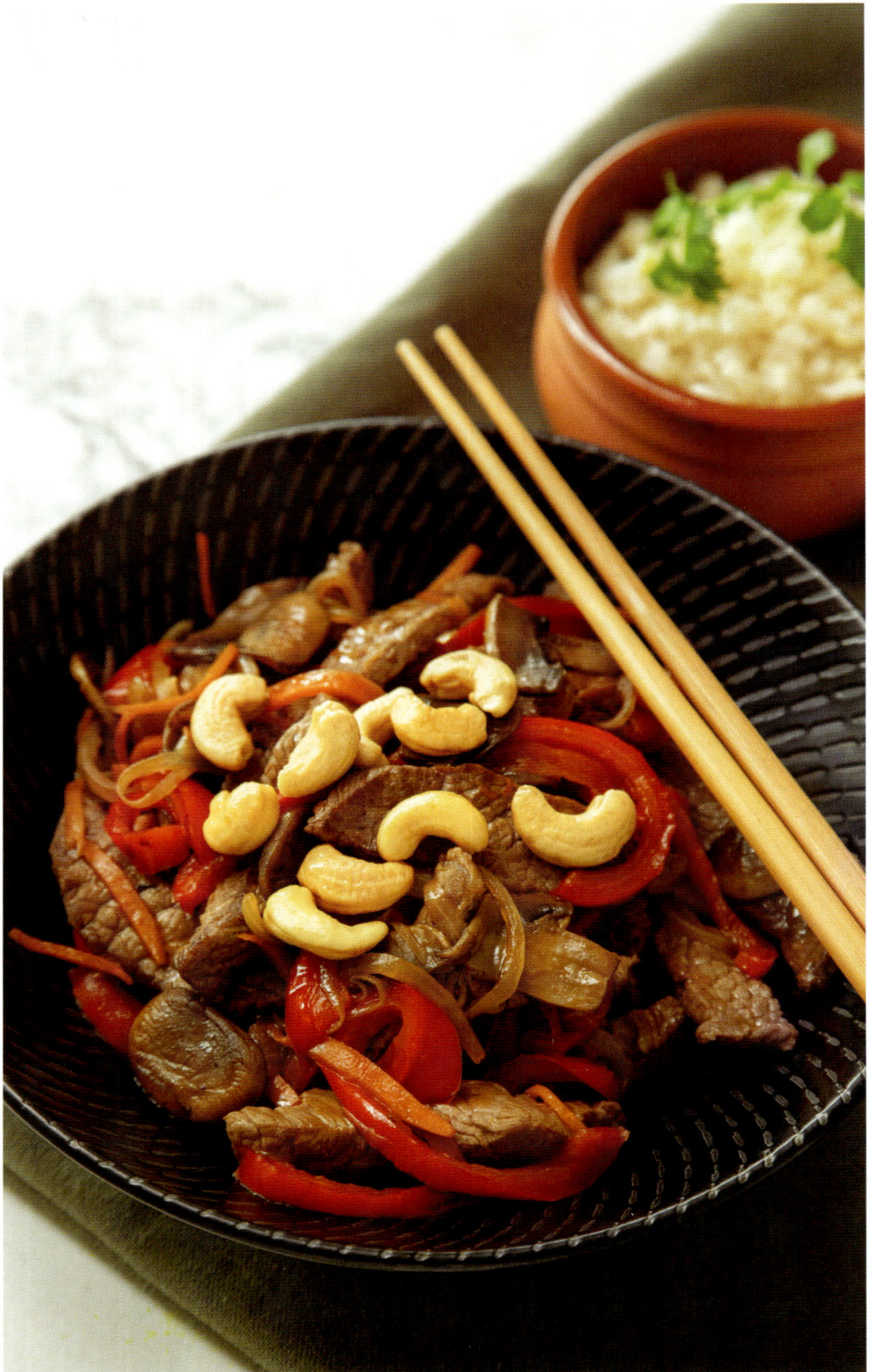

Capsicum Beef Stir-fry with Cauli Rice, page 255

EXAMPLES OF PHYSICAL HUNGER	EXAMPLES OF HEAD HUNGER
Often builds slowly over time.	Often comes out of nowhere.
3–4 hours have passed since you last ate.	Minimal time has passed; often you feel hungry just after you ate.
You can often wait a little longer to eat if you really need to.	A strong desire to eat the food right now; there's a lot of urgency attached to eating.
Happy to eat any type of food including healthy foods.	Often crave a specific food, e.g. something sweet only.
Your body responds to the hunger, e.g. rumbling tummy, feeling low in energy.	You're experiencing a large emotion, e.g. very stressed, sad, lonely.
You feel satisfied after eating.	Often once you eat the food you craved, you crave more and you are rarely satisfied from just a small amount.
After eating you can happily move on without any guilt or resentment.	Often there are feelings of regret or guilt after eating.

Non-hunger-based eating poses issues when it comes to weight control, and even more so if the goal is fat loss. While there are some people who genuinely do not feel hunger and need to eat to plan, for the average person, if we eat when we are not hungry, ultimately we will be consuming calories we do not need. This leaves us prone to gradually increasing weight gain over time, or in real-life terms, an extra kilo or two each year we barely notice until it is more like 5 or 10 kilos and much harder to lose.

Now we are not saying that you can never eat if you are feeling head hungry as a large part of our life is based around celebrating or rewarding with food. But if you can tune into your body and appreciate when it isn't truly hungry, portions at these celebrations can become smaller and you can learn to adjust the next meal or snack, if needed, which will also help with weight control longer term.

The other issue with non-hunger-based eating is that over time we become less and less aware of our natural hunger and fullness signals, and even uncomfortable with experiencing any degree of hunger, so we might tend to eat to avoid becoming hungry at all. This leaves us in a constant state of overeating and requires significant reprogramming so we can get back in touch with our hunger and learn to optimally regulate our appetite again.

NOTES FROM THE NUTRITION COUCH
TIPS FOR DEALING WITH EMOTIONAL EATING

When we emotionally eat, we tend to confuse our feelings with physical hunger cues. If you feel the need to emotionally eat, there are some strategies to help manage it that can be easily added to your routine.

1. **Understand**: Just like we discussed in Chapter 1, emotional eating can stem from childhood experiences with food. It can be as simple as having seen that behaviour modelled to us by our parents. There may be issues in our lives that contribute to the habit.
2. **Write it down**: Keeping a journal can help our brains identify common threads that lead to emotional eating. Journalling your emotions is also a good strategy to help you identify and prioritise problems, fears and concerns. Journalling emotions and symptoms regularly can help you recognise triggers and learn other coping strategies.
3. **Change the environment**: From what you may have discovered by understanding the causes of your emotional eating and writing down how you feel when you do it, you can help yourself avoid the temptation in future. For example, you may find you are likely to emotionally eat in front of the TV after a long day at work. Instead, try eating a snack at the dining table with no distractions.

10 October 2021[79]

Tune back into your natural hunger

The first step in taking back control of your natural hunger is to start to assess it. The busy nature of modern life means that we are often eating on autocue rather than because we are truly hungry. Eating can also be a welcome relief from the mundane nature of daily life, but constant snacking and grazing throughout the day can mean we never have the 3 to 4 hours in between meals without food to fully digest all the food in the stomach and subsequently experience natural hunger come a mealtime. And if you are someone who has a history of yo-yo dieting, it may be possible that over the years, you have learnt to ignore the hunger signals your body sends out.

To help tune back in, pay attention to your appetite at a mealtime and give it a rating out of 10 to help quantify it. While the goal is not to wait until you are ravenous before eating, most of the time we eat when we are feeling a 4 to 5 out of 10 hunger-wise, versus the 7 to 8 we ideally should be. Sometimes you will find it is okay to wait an hour or two to eat at a time when you feel truly hungry, rather than eating because other people are, or because it is a mealtime. While it is ideal to wait until you are hungry to eat a meal, if you are someone who never really feels hungry, especially in the morning, it can be better to eat something small within an hour or two of waking, to help stimulate metabolism and get the digestive system working, especially if you are out of the habit of eating breakfast.

If you do not tend to wake up hungry this could be for a few reasons. Milky drinks, including both coffee and tea, can displace morning hunger. We should experience natural hunger 3 to 4 hours after breakfast; however, if you're drinking a few of these across the morning you will sip on your calories over several hours rather than enjoying a balanced meal. This may have a knock-on effect of causing you to overeat during the afternoon and evening because you've kept hunger at bay until lunchtime. Eating late at night can also displace morning hunger, especially if you find you are eating heavier meals and having less than 12 hours overnight without food.

If you don't experience any hunger within an hour or two of waking:

- Try having your dinner earlier – make sure you finish eating by 8 pm each night at the latest.
- Focus on eating lighter meals at night rather than consuming your largest meal of the day then.
- To give your metabolism a kickstart, within an hour or two of waking eat a small breakfast of protein and carbohydrates, such as a slice of toast with an egg or Greek yoghurt with fruit.
- Try shifting all your meals an hour earlier to wake up your metabolism.
- Keep an eye on milk-based coffees, which can depress appetite through the morning.
- You can also try some morning exercise to stimulate your hunger.

Identify your hunger

If you find yourself feeling the urge to eat something outside of a mealtime, pause for a moment and work out what kind of hunger it is that you're feeling. Are you feeling bored or tired? Are you holding negative emotions and looking for comfort and pleasure in food? Have you left it too long since you last ate so now you're over-hungry and feel like your blood sugar is low? Rather than snacking, do you instead need to eat a properly balanced meal? Once you're clear on what's driving your desire to eat and why, this can help you redirect and take alternative action that's likely to be much better for your mind and body.

WHAT TYPE OF HUNGRY ARE YOU?	TIPS FOR MANAGING
Head hungry	Distract yourself – do something to take your focus off food.
Emotionally hungry	Look for other ways to self-soothe, e.g. a bath, massage, calling a friend or exercise.
Tired hungry	Revitalise with a cup of tea or coffee, some fresh air or gentle stretching.
Over-hungry	Seek out a balanced meal to satisfy yourself rather than overeating snack food.
Bored hungry	Change your environment and go do something immersive.

What if I am constantly hungry?

If you feel as though you are always hungry, there are a few reasons why this may be happening:

- It may be that not all of what you're sensing is true, physical hunger. Some could be head hunger, as discussed above – see if you can attribute it to any of those other causes.
- Perhaps your meals aren't high volume enough to keep you satisfied for several hours, in which case you need to bulk them up with more vegetables/salads (more on this in Chapter 9).
- Maybe your diet doesn't feature enough fibre. Without adequate fibre, you will feel hunger sooner and are more likely to struggle with digestive issues as well. As we saw in the previous chapter, fibre is a magical nutrient that allows the body to feel fuller for longer as it helps to slow the digestion of food in our stomach.
- We often find that clients who are constantly hungry aren't balancing their meals properly. The meals often lack an important macronutrient component such as carbohydrates or protein, so clients feel hungrier sooner. A well-balanced meal should keep us full and satisfied for several hours after eating.

- If your meals are well balanced, perhaps you simply aren't eating enough, particularly if you are quite active or living in a larger body. Eating 20 to 30 per cent more at mealtimes when your meals are well balanced is a far better strategy than over-snacking between mealtimes.

Hormones can affect appetite

Another common reason you may not be feeling hungry or feel hungry all the time is because of hormonal issues. Fat metabolism and appetite regulation involve a number of hormones including ghrelin, leptin, cortisol and oestrogen, and the glucose-management hormone we met earlier, insulin. It is common to see these disrupted in people with obesity.[80]

In particular, dysfunctional insulin impacts where we store body fat, how well we metabolise glucose from carbohydrates, the amount of insulin released when we eat, and how effectively our muscles can burn stored fat. If you are eating well and exercising yet are still struggling to lose weight, especially around the abdominal area, this may be suggestive of potential insulin- and glucose-regulation issues that should be medically investigated.

Equally, it may point towards the effects of your changing hormones through peri-menopause – the period of 2 to 10 years in which your body gets ready for menopause. During peri-menopause, the hormone oestrogen starts to decline, kickstarting a follow-on effect for metabolism and abdominal weight gain. During these years many women may experience central weight gain, which can exacerbate underlying insulin issues should they be present. Ultimately this can make weight loss challenging and can also increase the risk of developing type 2 diabetes.

While declining oestrogen is normal, working to actively prevent the weight gain associated with this is crucial if you are in peri-menopause. Here, reducing calorie and carbohydrate intake slightly, plus committing to resistance training at least twice each week can help to buffer the impact of declining oestrogen levels and help keep you in control of your weight.

SIGNS YOU MAY HAVE A HORMONAL IMBALANCE

Symptoms caused by hormone imbalances include low mood, extreme fatigue, extreme irritability, out-of-control hunger or lack of hunger, poor sleep and unexplained weight loss or gain. If you're experiencing any of these symptoms or if you have tried to reprogram your hunger without success, or cannot get control over your hunger, it may be time to see a doctor for support in managing your hormones and/or a dietitian to look at options that could help with glucose regulation and appetite management.

Mindful eating

Whether it's a few too many cocktails on a Friday night, that extra row of chocolate after dinner or a cheeky cake when you have a coffee with your friend, a 'treat' can be something that slips into the diet on more days than not and quickly becomes a calorie overload. We all have our things – be they chocolate, cheese, chips or anything else – but ultimately these high-calorie foods need to be proactively managed when your goal is fat loss.

While there is nothing wrong with any of these foods in isolation, it is their calorie density that poses an issue when you are actively trying to create and maintain a calorie deficit. Consider that a single small glass of wine or a typical row of chocolate contains more than 100 calories. Eating just one or two serves of 'extra', discretionary calories each day can therefore negate fat loss, making it difficult to achieve your weight-loss goals. If you're serious about fat loss you need to get honest and serious about how and when you include these foods in your diet, and not let them make regular appearances.

Enjoying more indulgent foods occasionally is absolutely fine – you'll certainly never hear us say you cannot enjoy a meal out, dessert or your favourite treat. Instead, the key to achieving fat loss and weight control while still eating these foods is to work out what the right *balance* is for you. For example, are you someone who can enjoy an individual chocolate or a single glass of wine every day without being tempted to keep indulging? Or, do you know you need to limit these foods and only have them occasionally as you find it difficult to control yourself? Do you prefer to eat strictly during the week, so that you can relax a little on the weekend? Every person is different and there is not a one-size-fits-all model. When limitations are externally imposed on individuals, they're rarely sustainable. The best dietary pattern for you is one that you have agency to direct and control, and one that you genuinely like. It's as simple as that.

Treats can be considered in two ways. The first is a genuine 'treat' such as finding yourself at a special restaurant or celebration and genuinely enjoying a special food that you would not usually consume. Here you are consuming a meal or special foods as part of an event or celebration, which is a completely normal part of life and something we both do and encourage. Life is too short not to eat some delicious dessert at a special restaurant! However, the most important thing to note here is the quality of the food. There's a big difference between the mass-produced supermarket office biscuits that are always available and the very special chef-created chocolate torte with quality ingredients that you have never tried before.

The second way we would classify a treat is the more frequently mentioned daily 'treat'. These often slip in mindlessly when we are offered foods by others, or come with a degree of entitlement whereby, just because we *feel* like eating something we think we *should* be allowed to, or we are rewarding ourselves in some way with food. The trick is not to avoid treats altogether, but consider how they can fit into weight management.

NOTES FROM THE NUTRITION COUCH
5 NON-NEGOTIABLE DAILY ACTIONS FOR GOOD HEALTH

1. **Check in with your goals**: Spend 5, 10 or 30 minutes focusing on what you want to achieve each day. It doesn't need to be a meditation session; instead, try to fit it into your daily life. For example, you could do this while you're taking your dog for a walk or grocery shopping.

2. **Get moving**: Any kind of movement or exercise for 20 minutes a day will do wonders for your mental and physical wellbeing, and it doesn't have to mean going to the gym. You could do some stretching after putting the kids to bed, or even do some squats while supervising their time at the playground.

3. **Eat your meals mindfully**: Sit down to enjoy your food without distractions and pay attention to what you are eating. This not only helps with digestion but helps your brain register fullness and can prevent overeating.

4. **Prioritise 5 veg, 2 fruit serves**: It may seem like common sense, but getting in as many nutrients from fresh foods as possible is an actionable step that can make a sustained difference to your health. Focus on what you can add into your diet, not on what you need to cut out.

5. **Get in touch with your emotions**: We all live busy lives and can run on autopilot, but if you sit down and do some deep breathing or journalling it can set you up for success in the long term.

24 May 2023[81]

Enjoy your favourite foods mindfully

Savouring good quality food with friends and family is one of life's most simple pleasures, and as such, you should never skip the special meal or birthday cake to self-punish. If you cognitively control your food intake this way, eventually resentment tends to build and you are more likely to overeat tempting foods when you cease the self-imposed rules that stop you from eating foods that you usually would in a given situation.

A much healthier, more sustainable mindset when it comes to treats is to ask yourself a few questions:

1. Is it really a special occasion?
2. Is the food really top quality or just run of the mill?
3. Are you truly hungry? Do you need a whole piece or will just a little taste satisfy?
4. Do you honestly feel like and want the particular food that's on offer?

The key here is to pause, break that auto-response circuit and really take some time to reflect on what you genuinely feel like eating when faced with more calorie-dense foods. Many of us, especially those with a long history of dieting, have been programmed to eat on autocue, grabbing 'junk' and discretionary foods whenever we have access or permission to eat them, regardless of whether we want or like what we are eating. We eat quickly, barely noticing the tastes or flavours of what we are consuming, which ultimately leads to overeating. Simply slowing down can be enough to shift your eating from autocue to mindfulness.

When you do choose to eat and enjoy a more indulgent food, no matter what it may be, it is incredibly important to take the time to identify what will bring you the most satisfaction. Often when you pause to understand what you really want, you'll find that it's not in fact the 'bad' food you were about to eat simply because it was available. In many cases, when we look at and properly consider our food choices in this way, we also find that we need much less of the indulgent food to feel satisfied. Often the foods don't taste as good as they look and after a bite or two, you are happy to leave it.

To reach this stage of self-regulated food intake is incredibly empowering and ultimately enables you to control your weight for life. Here there are no foods you can't eat. Instead, it's about asking yourself what you really feel like eating and, once you start to eat, whether it actually tastes good. In this way, you are able to take or leave it with full control and peace of mind.

For those who have restricted their food intake for some time, you can imagine this can take some practice to master – but it's definitely possible. The first step is simply checking in and considering what you really feel like eating. Then eating mindfully – without distraction, not in front of the TV, but with focus on your food. Chew carefully; really experience the flavours and textures so that you're more attuned to the tastes of the food you are eating and how much you are enjoying eating it. Don't be afraid to stop eating or put the food down if it simply isn't as satisfying as you thought it would be.

A classic example to demonstrate this is when we are offered birthday cake at work. Typically, you may have taken it and eaten it quickly, perhaps while chatting to a colleague or sitting in front of your computer, not fully registering it. If, instead, you eat slowly and mindfully, in many cases you may either find the cake is not that great at all, or that after a mouthful or two you've had enough and can leave the rest. You do not have to eat everything you are served. On the other hand, refusing the cake but then sneaking back several times to grab a spoonful or two when no one else is looking kind of defeats the purpose, yet is incredibly common for those who have previously been on restrictive diets.

If you know that you need some help in this area, start by differentiating special-occasion foods such as restaurant meals or desserts from the run-of-the mill treats that can slip into your day, such as biscuits at work or fundraising chocolates. Keeping your high-calorie treat intake controlled and limited to special occasions when you enjoy such special foods mindfully will help to make it easier to say no when routine extras are offered to you day-to-day.

In the case of more indulgent meals or occasions that come with lots of extra calories – weekends away, restaurant meals, celebrations – very few of us can get away with eating like this more than once a week and still lose body fat. At best, this type of over-consumption will result in reaching a weight plateau. This often happens when you find yourself in situations where there are several higher calorie meals in a short period of time. So, bear in mind that while you can buffer these occasions somewhat by eating less for a day or two, or exercising more, they will certainly make fat loss much more difficult.

How to incorporate small daily treats

With all that said, we know from our client work that including those indulgent foods you really enjoy eating can play a helpful part in long-term weight management. Diet plans become a lot more appealing when they include the foods you love eating every day. Within a calorie-controlled eating plan, factoring in a small number of calories each day that are dedicated to more indulgent foods tends to aid dietary compliance, as you are less likely to feel deprived long term.

When you take a closer look at calorie loads, and even calorie intake recommendations that support sustainable fat loss, there is generally room for an extra 'treat' or some 'soul food' each day – something that clocks in around 100 calories, such as a small glass of wine with dinner, or a 100-calorie dessert to end the day's eating.

TIPS FOR INCLUDING SMALL TREATS THAT DON'T SABOTAGE YOUR FAT-BURNING GOALS

- Try to avoid eating food and snacks on the run. Making it a priority to sit down and enjoy balanced meals will go a long way towards keeping your calorie intake controlled. We understand that sometimes this isn't practical but, on the whole, aim to eat the majority of meals and snacks as mindfully as possible so the brain has time to appreciate that you've eaten.

For example, sip on a glass of wine slowly to fully savour the experience, or follow dinner with a Lindt ball at the table and fully enjoy over several minutes without the distraction of the TV.

- Take time to consider what it is you really feel like – is it a piece of chocolate, or some ice-cream? Or are you looking for something salty or crunchy? Identifying what will bring you the most satisfaction will aid mindful eating. Make your treat count!

- Impose a general guideline of limiting the intake of sweet foods until after dinner. This will help make it easier to say no to the little extras that can slip into our day, like a biscuit, cake or chocolate at work each afternoon. Avoiding sweet food throughout the day will also help support blood-glucose control and prevent cravings. Often, eating sweet foods early in the day piques our cravings and it becomes harder to say no to more sweet foods later on.

- Ultimately, the key is portion control, so opt for foods you will not overeat and help yourself by purchasing individual portions of treats rather than large packets or tubs. Another trick is to opt for stronger flavours to help aid satisfaction – think higher percentage dark chocolate, or a piece of mature cheese.

- Stop at one. As noted above, when the goal is fat loss there is generally room in your overall daily intake for one small treat but no more, so make your selection for the day, enjoy it, and remember there is always tomorrow to enjoy the next one.

Take control of the weekends

When it comes to fat loss, weekends are tricky. The days are less structured, there is often plenty of socialising, eating out and celebratory meals that include alcohol, kids' sport and travel – as well as a general desire to stop any strict program or diet and enjoy the food and drink on offer. The issue with a typical free-flowing weekend is that it can result in hundreds of extra calories being consumed, which certainly impacts fat loss.

The key to not undoing an entire week of hard work is to plan out the weekend so that you can identify which meals may be considered 'special', for example a birthday or event, versus the run-of-the-mill scenarios like bacon and eggs rolls at the rugby or grabbing takeaway, which you can maintain a lot more control over.

Throughout the course of a weekend, from a calorie perspective, you can factor in a meal or two that is more indulgent and still keep your fat-loss goals on track if you maintain your dietary balance and structure the remainder of the time. Weekends may also mean that you need fewer meals, as some may be larger. Or you may have a lighter meal or two to compensate for more indulgent, higher calorie meals out or several alcoholic drinks. For example, enjoying a later, larger brunch on a Sunday, followed by a light afternoon snack and a light soup or protein-rich salad for dinner may help to buffer the extras that can slip in as part of a regular weekend.

Ultimately, keeping in control on the weekends will come down to planning – proactively setting aside time each week to map out the weekend and identify when you will indulge and when you will need to prep and plan your food in advance to keep things on track.

Enjoy a food-friendly life

Learning what to eat and how to nourish our bodies is key to good nutrition. In the earlier chapters we reset our mindset and built our knowledge around solid nutrition guidelines, so we know better what to eat. Now that we've learnt to tune into our natural hunger signals and embrace them as a friendly ally in our bid for sustainable weight loss while enjoying the occasional treat, let's turn our attention to how best to time our meals.

CHAPTER 8

TIME YOUR MEALS

We were once told that it does not matter *when* you consume your calories and as long as you do not consume more than you need, you will not gain weight. Science now tells us this is not always the case. Meal timing matters, especially when it comes to metabolic health and weight control.[82]

Put simply, the human body is programmed to a circadian rhythm or 24-hour clock that directs it to move and burn calories throughout the day and store excess energy at night. This is due to the hormones that control fat metabolism and energy regulation, and the general fact that we tend to be more active in the day. While it's not impossible to work against this inbuilt clock, as many shift workers and international jetsetters must do, it does make it harder to manage weight and fatigue (particularly as you get older) since you're working against the body's natural rhythms.[83]

In practical terms this means that if you routinely eat very little through the morning, instead relying on coffee and snacks before overeating throughout the afternoon and evening, weight loss will be challenging no matter how many calories you consume. But if you know how to balance your meals well across the day, to shift your calories forward and support natural metabolic function, you'll ultimately be supporting weight control.

While we may often hear about macros and calories, the reality is that we eat food as meals and snacks. For this reason, describing nutritional balance in terms of meal structure makes sense, especially when it comes to working towards a balance for fat loss. In this chapter we'll cover not just when to eat, but what to eat at different times of day to achieve the right balance.

Meet Nikita: feeling the benefits of balanced eating ⌂

At 52 years old, Nikita found herself in a quieter new chapter, with the youngest of her children having moved out to begin university. With newfound time to focus on herself, she set some ambitious lifestyle goals: to cultivate stable energy throughout the day, tame her sugar cravings, lose 7 kilograms and run a half marathon in 6 months.

When Nikita went for her first consultation with her dietitian, she explained that she had been doing intermittent fasting for a couple of years in the hope of managing her weight, and would fast from 8 pm until noon the next day. During the mornings she would consume 3 cups of black coffee but while those offered a temporary lift, she'd feel her energy levels crashing by midday. When she finally ate her meals were large and laden with refined carbs – white bread, sushi rolls and creamy pasta – foods that delivered short-lived fullness but gave way to hunger pangs soon after.

She would exercise on an empty stomach and then resist the urge to refuel, despite her body's protests of hunger. This pattern led to a cycle of over-indulgence during her eating window, as she sought to satisfy her hunger with heavy, filling meals that ultimately sabotaged her weight-loss efforts. Her diet, low in protein and fibre and devoid of vegetables, left her blood sugars on a rollercoaster and her cravings uncontrolled.

Nikita's journey to transformation required a rethink of how she timed her meals across the day. It began with a pivotal shift: she gave up the intermittent fasting and introduced a balanced breakfast, sprinkled with cinnamon for its blood-sugar–regulating properties. She began to honour her body's need for fuel, having a small snack on training days before her morning gym session and following up with a nutritious breakfast within an hour of finishing her training. She added milk to her mid-morning coffee to increase her protein and calcium intake and her satiety. Nikita's approach to coffee changed in other ways, too; she started drinking it *after* food to aid in stress regulation.

To add much-needed bulk and nutrients to her meals, Nikita made cooked vegetables a staple in her lunches and dinners, as she preferred them over salad. Whole grains were woven into her diet to increase her fibre intake, assist with blood-sugar regulation and distribute her carbohydrate consumption more evenly throughout the day.

The outcome of these strategic changes was profound. Nikita's energy levels stabilised, her digestion improved, she performed better in her training and her sleep became more restful. She no longer felt overstuffed at bedtime, which contributed to better sleep quality. Her cravings subsided as her meals became more balanced, and she was more attuned to her body's hunger and fullness signals.

After 4 months of dedication to her new lifestyle, Nikita not only reached but surpassed her weight-loss goal, shedding 7.3 kilograms. Her training paid off spectacularly when she crossed the finish line of her half marathon having run the whole way, setting a personal best in the process. Nikita had redefined her relationship with food and exercise, moving from a cycle of fasting and feasting to a balanced, better-timed approach that supported her body's needs and her athletic ambitions.

Metabolism-boosting mornings

While every day is different, as a rule of thumb, the earlier you have your first meal the better it is for metabolic rate. The human body is naturally programmed according to circadian rhythms, setting our hormones and digestive system to work during the day, and to rest and replenish at night. Eating something early, within an hour or so of waking, helps to stoke the metabolic fire and gets the body busy burning calories. It's also beneficial from a digestive-health perspective to factor in a 10- to 12-hour window without eating overnight, so for most people this will mean eating their first meal between 6 am and 9 am each day.

If you are one of the many people who do not feel hungry in the morning, this is likely a result of overeating at night or being in the habit of not eating until later in the day, or both. While it is always ideal to feel hungry before eating, in this instance, starting to eat something small within an hour or two of waking will retrain your metabolism over time to get burning earlier in the day. Once you become aware of this hunger, you can then time your subsequent meals accordingly.

Sometimes we find people avoid eating breakfast as they find it makes them hungrier throughout the day. While eating earlier in the day may give you a metabolic boost resulting in increases in appetite, the key to managing this is to ensure your meal choices are high in protein, fibre and volume to help keep you full and satisfied for several hours. If you keep in mind that from a metabolic perspective regular hunger is a good thing, experiencing it will not be so disconcerting.

The ingredients of a great breakfast

Long gone are the days when families would sit together and discuss the day ahead over a bowl of cereal and homemade coffee. Nowadays, breakfast is more likely to be a takeaway coffee or croissant enjoyed on the go, or shifted to a late-morning brunch or early lunch as intermittent fasting has become increasingly popular.

While the importance of breakfast has been downplayed for many, the reality is that eating a nutrient-rich meal within an hour or two of waking has several metabolic benefits. A nutritionally balanced breakfast will contain a mix of protein, wholegrains and good fats from fresh food to help create a meal that will keep you full and satisfied for several hours; a meal that will support blood-glucose control and offer a range of key essential nutrients including dietary fibre, calcium, iron and zinc. Good protein-rich foods include eggs, smoked salmon, yoghurt, milk, cottage cheese or protein-based breads and cereals. Wholegrains from grain and seeded breads and cereals, and legumes and fresh foods including fruit and vegetables that can be enjoyed with eggs or blended into smoothies and juices are all good options. A source of good fat, via avocado, nuts or seeds, will to add to the nutritional profile of your breakfast.

TOP NUTRIENT-RICH BREAKFASTS

- Eggs and veggies on wholegrain toast.
- Breakfast smoothie with added protein, e.g. Greek yoghurt or protein powder, and added fats such as almond butter – try our Banana and Almond Smoothie (page 239).
- Baked oats served with a high-protein yoghurt and fruit.
- Overnight oats or bircher made with seeds, milk, berries and Greek yoghurt – try our Overnight Berry Bircher (page 240).
- Low-sugar, wholegrain cereal with milk and nuts/seeds.
- Baked beans on grain toast.
- Cottage cheese and roasted vegetables on wholegrain toast.
- Mexican Eggs with Beans (page 241) or bean shakshuka with vegetables.
- Salad and smoked salmon grain wrap.
- Avocado and tomato on high-protein toast or wholegrain toast.

- Breakfast Nourish Bowl (page 242) with Greek yoghurt and some healthy fats.
- Egg and vegetable frittata with added potato or sweet potato.
- Chia pudding made with a protein source such as Greek yoghurt or protein powder.
- Vegetable Egg Bites (page 238) served with eggs and avocado.

If a cooked breakfast seems overwhelming on a busy workday, save it for the weekend or a day off when you have a little more time. For the busy workdays use some meal-prep options like overnight oats, egg bites or smoothies, which can be pre-made and packed up so you're ready to go in the morning in a matter of minutes.

What about coffee?

The popularity of milk-based coffees like lattes and cappuccinos to start the day is a factor to consider when getting your breakfast balance right. While a milk-based coffee does contain calories (anywhere from 60 to 150 calories depending on size), it is certainly not a breakfast substitute. But a milk coffee to start the day can significantly impact appetite, pushing your first meal or real hunger until mid-to-late morning.

If you love a milk coffee to start the day, it is much better to team it with a small breakfast and complete the meal, or opt for black tea or coffee first, before adding a milk coffee to your breakfast meal, rather than sipping on milk-based coffee over a period of time. This ensures your mealtimes are isolated and allows for at least 2 to 3 hours in between meals for blood glucose and digestive hormones to return to baseline levels. This is important for both weight control and hunger management, especially with hormonal-type conditions. If you are someone who struggles with stress, high cortisol or anxiety, you may find that having your coffee with food rather than on an empty stomach helps control your symptoms better.[84]

Should I eat morning tea?

Grabbing a snack mid-to-late morning regardless of appetite is a relatively common habit. The issue with snacking when it is closer to lunch than breakfast is that lunch tends to get pushed back to as late as 2 or 3 pm, shifting calorie intake into the second half of the day. For most people who have eaten breakfast at 7 or 8 am, having an early lunch is a better option for metabolism and weight control.

In saying that, for individuals who are up early every day, who are training early or who are not actively trying to lose weight, if you are genuinely hungry 2 to 3 hours after breakfast and it is only 10 am, a protein-rich morning tea can be a good idea. Make a nutritionally balanced choice such as a Greek yoghurt with fruit and nuts, or cheese and crackers, which will keep you satisfied for another couple of hours. Not only should you steer away from pastries but also most sweet snacks including regular muesli bars, muffins, fruit yoghurts and biscuits – they will drive appetite and cravings plus largely lack the nutritional balance of a satisfying snack.

NOTES FROM THE NUTRITION COUCH
HOW TO MANAGE BREAKFAST TIME AND HUNGER LEVELS

Ultimately, the best indicator of when you should eat, and how much, is your hunger level. Breakfast is the ideal time to tune in to this. We know that breakfast can help stabilise blood-sugar levels, give us a necessary burst of energy and sustain focus and productivity. Regular eating in the morning also helps our hunger levels align with our circadian rhythm.

Scenario 1: Waking up and not feeling hungry
Try eating half the portion size of your normal breakfast. This way, you're not skipping the meal entirely and are still starting the day with some nutrients.

> **Scenario 2: Waking up hungrier than usual**
> Give yourself permission to eat more. It may seem almost con-
> fronting to trust your hunger levels, but listening to what your body
> needs will pay dividends throughout the day. Some days the body
> is just hungrier than other days, and this is perfectly okay as you
> may also find that on other days you're *less* hungry.
>
> *8 October 2023*[85]

Let's talk about . . . intermittent fasting

There has been a lot of hype around intermittent fasting over the
past 5 to 10 years, so let's separate facts from fancy. Intermittent
fasting is when you cycle between periods of fasting and periods
of eating using variable meal timings. There are many types of
fasting including time-restricted fasting,. periodic fasting or
alternate-day fasting. Some of the more popular fasting protocols
you may have heard of are the 5:2 diet and the 16:8 method.

The primary reason intermittent fasting can assist with weight
loss is due to an overall reduction in calories thanks to a reduced
time of eating. Sadly, weight loss is not a benefit everyone sees
as it is very easy to overeat your calories even in a smaller eating
window. Therefore, your diet quality and exercise regimen still
matter, whether using intermittent fasting or not.

While for some people this approach works really well, there
is nothing magical about intermittent fasting from a fat-loss perspective. Sure, your body enters a fat-burning state after it has
used the calories from the meals consumed, but the body can also
do this without fasting if you are eating in a calorie deficit. Why
fasting seems to work for many people is that entering this state of
reduced calories is easier when you can skip a meal or two.

As well as the weight-related benefits, some research also
points towards fasting helping with blood pressure and blood

sugar control, as well as assisting with brain health and helping to repair damaged cells.[86] It may also assist with some digestive concerns as you are giving the gut time to 'rest and digest'.[87]

If you find fasting easy and beneficial for you, by all means use it, but if you feel like it creates too much rigidity or negative thinking around food, you may want eat more regularly. If you find you overeat at mealtimes, feel too full when you are going to bed, or have troubles making progress with your training efforts, you may want to rethink fasting as a tool for you.

GROUPS OF PEOPLE FOR WHOM INTERMITTENT FASTING IS NOT RECOMMENDED

- Pregnant or breastfeeding women.
- Those under 18 or over 70.
- Those with an eating disorder or history of one.
- Those with already restrictive eating patterns.
- Those who have issues with blood-sugar regulation, low blood pressure or who often feel light-headed.
- Athletes or those who exercise at a higher level or more than once a day.
- Those with higher requirements, e.g. someone undergoing cancer treatment.
- Those whose medication is reliant on being taken with food.

Other medical strategies for weight management

With diabetes and its comorbidity of obesity on the rise globally, there are several treatment pathways being trialled and investigated, including fasting, as described above, bariatric surgery and drug interventions.[88] Recent breakthrough semaglutide weight-loss drugs, branded under such recognisable names as Ozempic and Wegovy, have gained a serious following.

In terms of weight-loss drugs, these semaglutides are unique as they not only help to regulate appetite, but also help to stimulate insulin production in the pancreas. For individuals with blood-glucose regulation issues, as is the case in insulin resistance and type 2 diabetes, these drugs can significantly reduce appetite. This aids calorie-controlled eating, while also increasing the body's ability to reduce insulin levels, ultimately supporting fat loss.

For individuals who have had high insulin for some time and have had a lot of difficulty losing weight, these drugs can be revolutionary, but they require just as much attention to diet and exercise – if not more – to yield large results long term. For this reason, many people who do get results using these drugs also fail in their attempts, simply because they have not made sustainable changes to their diet and exercise habits.

Nothing will command a headline like a new weight-loss drug, and while there have been several of these drugs introduced over the past 20 years, the reality is that none of them holds the key to weight loss. At best they can make dietary compliance easier and support weight loss, but there are none you can take and expect to be kilos lighter without also following through with a serious lifestyle change.[89]

HOW DO I KNOW IF I MAY NEED MEDICATION TO SUPPORT WEIGHT LOSS?

If any of the following are true for you, it may be time to have a consultation with your GP or endocrinologist to see if there are any signs of hormonal dysfunction that may be impacting your weight:

- You have a family history of type 2 diabetes.
- You've had gestational diabetes.

- You have other autoimmune diseases and/or they run in the family, e.g. thyroid dysfunction.[90]
- You have a waist measurement above 90 centimetres.
- You are more than 10 kilograms overweight and have difficulty losing weight no matter what you do.

The important thing to keep in mind is that while short-term weight loss can be achieved through a variety of modalities, medicines included, long-term maintenance is much more challenging. To sustain weight loss over the long term, a permanent lifestyle shift to a healthy diet and regular exercise regimen is ultimately the key.[91]

Give lunch more attention

If we were to deem one meal more important than the others for overall food balance, it would be lunch, though it's not always given the focus it deserves. Nutritionally, this meal plays a major role in regulating food intake and eating behaviour throughout the afternoon and evening. Not only is a well-timed lunch crucial to optimally fuel the body for the afternoon, but a well-balanced lunch will assist in stabilising blood-glucose levels and help you to avoid sweet cravings come later afternoon.

As we learnt earlier, meal timing matters, as we can use our circadian rhythm to our advantage. If you do eat late in the day or too many hours after your first meal, you will fail to tap into the metabolic boost we naturally get during the first half of the day. Therefore, the earlier you have your lunch, even in place of a late-morning snack, the better it will be for fat burning.

If you are hungry at 11 am or 11.30 am, eat your lunch then. If you hold off, filling the gap with a snack instead, only to have a late lunch and more sweet foods at 3 or 4 pm, your blood glucose is more likely to have dropped significantly, leaving you ravenous and prone to overeating.

Think back to a time when you have enjoyed a filling, large lunch . . . remember the way you did not find yourself searching for snacks all afternoon, and didn't even really feel like dinner? A well-balanced, nutritious, hearty lunch meal enjoyed earlier in the day will not only help keep you full and satisfied all afternoon but will also help you to get the protein and vegetable bulk you need to optimise your nutrient intake. It also sets you up for a lighter evening meal, which we'll get onto next – the two go hand in hand.

This simple shift to prioritising a filling lunch slightly earlier in the day will revolutionise your daily food intake.

Getting your lunch balance right

Too frequently in this modern life, lunch has become a high-carb, processed meal we grab on the run, or a small bite-sized meal built on the belief we should be seeking something 'light'. Sushi, wraps and snacks, and even so-called healthy soups or salad tend to lack the protein and veggie bulk of a well-balanced refuel. They leave us feeling unsatisfied and come mid-to-late afternoon we find ourselves ravenous. This drives us to snack throughout the afternoon and overeat later in the day.

This doesn't have to be the case. Achieving the right lunch balance to support weight control is relatively easy, once you know what to aim for. To keep full for 3 to 4 hours, each lunch meal should contain 1 serve (as a rough guides use the examples below) of each of the following:

- **vegetable bulk:** at least 2 to 3 cups of loose salad or 1 to 2 cups of dense vegetables.
- **protein:** palm-sized portion of canned tuna, lean chicken breast, beef, beans or tofu.
- **carbohydrate:** if your day is mostly sitting, around half to three-quarters of a cup, or if you're very active, 1 to 2 cups of wholefood carbs such as sweet potato, beans or brown rice.

In terms of bread or crackers the low range is 1 slice of bread or 3 to 4 wholegrain crackers, and the active range is 2 slices of bread and up to 8 crackers.

- **good fat**: a tablespoon of olive oil dressing, a small handful of nuts, or quarter of an avocado will help to slow your digestion after lunch and keep you fuller for longer.

WHAT ARE SOME GOOD LUNCH OPTIONS?

- Wraps and homemade sandwiches packed full of lean protein, healthy fats and salad/veggies.
- Nourishing soups or stews packed full of protein and good quality carbs.
- Frittatas or mini egg bites served with wholegrain toast to make a meal-prep-friendly option.
- Wholegrain crackers topped with tuna, cottage cheese or smoked salmon paired with lots of additional sliced veggies plus some avocado.
- Adding a soup or salad as a side dish to your lunch meal to build a more satisfying meal.
- If you find yourself out and about, some healthier convenience options include rice paper rolls, chicken strips, corn, cheese and salad, a piece of frittata or a filo pastry with salad, or a naked burrito bowl with chicken and beans.
- Leftovers make a great lunch option that's time-efficient and substantial – perhaps the leftovers from one of our dinner recipes at the back of the book.

Smart snacks

When it comes to snacking, every person is different but most people will need one or two snacks each day in between meals to keep their body adequately fuelled. If you consider that a meal will generally keep you full for 3 to 4 hours, then depending on how early you eat breakfast, the average person will need one or two snacks each day.

If your goal is fat loss, you may want to prioritise savoury snacks as these tend to keep cravings under control a little better, and you may want to plan your snacks in advance. In our experience, people tend to over-snack on high-carb options when they grab what is available and convenient at the time, and these often aren't choices that support fat loss or blood sugar control.

The key thing to remember when choosing a snack is that it should fill you up for 1 to 2 hours, and contain key nutrients such as protein and/or dietary fibre to help keep hunger at bay for a decent amount of time. A well-balanced snack should also contain some fresh food – think a piece of fruit or chopped vegetables – to go alongside some of these calorie-controlled, nutrient-dense options such as the examples in the box below.

OUR TOP 10 FILLING SNACKS

1. Nut-based snack bar.
2. 4 wholegrain crackers with cheese.
3. Medium skim latte.
4. 150 g Greek or high-protein yoghurt and berries.
5. 2 corn crackers with cottage cheese and cucumber.
6. Half a cup of steamed edamame beans.
7. 3 cups of air-popped popcorn.
8. Small/mini protein bar and a piece of fruit.
9. 2 rye crackers with goat's cheese and tomato.
10. Boiled egg with 2 tablespoons of hummus and vegetable sticks.

Go light at night

After a long day, it is not surprising that many of us look forward to sitting down to enjoy a nourishing meal. The problem is we generally end up eating too much for that time of day. Not only are we eating when we are usually most hungry, but when we add up the snacks we munch on before dinner, any alcohol we indulge in, the main meal itself and then the sweet treats we tend to enjoy afterwards, it is not uncommon to see clients who are consuming more than 1000 calories after 6 pm each day. All this combines to make it the heaviest meal of the day, not helped by the long-held idea that it should be our most substantial and by the fact it's often one that we have more time and focus to prepare. It is no wonder so many of us find it hard to fend off the kilos.

But, in fact, one of the most powerful things we can do for health, digestion and weight control is to eat an earlier dinner and keep the size and calorie content of the meal controlled. Large meals at night not only add a significant number of calories into the diet at the time of day when we are least active but also mean we are less likely to have a minimum 12-hour overnight fast, which has been shown to be beneficial for digestive health.[92]

A lighter evening meal means you are more likely to wake up the next day and feel hungry for a breakfast meal, plus eating light at night will help you to sleep better, thanks to improved digestive comfort and reduced risk of indigestion. It will also support weight loss, if that is your goal. Specifically, in the case of weight control, lighter, lower calorie meals support a calorie deficit and fat loss, but this is dependent on eating enough through the day so dinner can be a smaller meal.

Considering that there can be more than 6 hours between lunch and dinner, most of us will need some sort of fuel top-up mid-afternoon to avoid late-afternoon eating that will impact our dinner. This means enjoying a protein- and veggie-rich snack

3 to 4 hours after lunch to help prevent overeating at dinner and through the evening. We've shared our top filling snack suggestions in the box above.

So what does a light dinner look like? If you need some nourishing and family-friendly dinner choices to support weight management, look no further than our 10 favourite options below and the Burn recipes we've included later in the book.

Spaghetti bolognese packed with legumes

Pasta is always a family favourite meal but try to reduce the amount of mince used and throw in a tin or two of brown lentils to boost the overall fibre of the meal (and save you some money!). Ensure you pack as many veggies into the bolognese as possible and use a high-fibre pasta. If you have fussy kids who refuse veggies, one trick is to grate or chop them finely or, if needed, use a stick blender to blend them in, making them invisible. Alternatively, you could add a side salad to boost your intake of nutrient-rich carbohydrates.

Prawn and mango tacos

Prawns are a very lean protein source and often overlooked. Cook them up with a little garlic and serve with tacos and some veggies such as shredded red cabbage and baby spinach, cherry tomatoes, finely chopped celery, fresh mango, coriander and chilli. If you want to make this a lighter meal, alternate each taco shell with a lettuce leaf.

Homemade pizza

A healthy pizza comes down to the base and the toppings. Try to opt for a thinner base, use small amounts of lean protein and load up the veggies. Try to avoid high-fat toppings such as sausage, salami and bacon and go easy on the cheese. Make yours a lighter and more nourishing meal by serving your pizza slices with a nice side salad.

Crumbed fish and roasted vegetables

Making your own crumbed fish is ideal, but if you're busy and time poor, there are a range of wholemeal crumbed fish options at the supermarket that are quite good. Look for nutrition labels that show at least 60 per cent fish on them. While the oven is on, make sure you take advantage of that and cook some roasted veggies such as potato, pumpkin, zucchini, mushrooms and red capsicum to bulk out your plate and keep you feeling fuller.

Shepherd's pie

There's nothing quite as comforting as a shepherd's pie. Try to pack as many vegetables into your lean mince mixture as possible and top it with a mixed-vegetable mash (that is, a blend of potato, sweet potato and pumpkin) to increase the vegetable volume and variety even further. Don't forget the cheese on top, which aids in achieving satiety from your meal, and serve your piece with a big side salad to complement it.

Garlic chicken stir-fry

Stir-fries are quick and easy dinner options but be careful with bottled sauces as they can often pack a calorie and sodium punch. It is far more nourishing to make a simple stir-fry sauce yourself from a little low-sodium soy sauce, oyster sauce, ginger, garlic and chilli flakes. Try to serve the stir-fry with a higher fibre carbohydrate option such as quinoa. As a general guide for nourishment and health, the vegetable amount on your plate should be more than the carb amount.

Dumplings, edamame and greens

A quick scan of the nutritional labels at the supermarket can reveal some easy, nutritious dumplings the whole family will love. Try to choose a brand with a higher percentage of meat or other protein and no added MSG. Greens such as bok choy, broccolini, snow peas and zucchini pair wonderfully with dumplings. Serving with a side of edamame can provide a great boost of carbs and fibre while still keeping the meal light.

Salmon nourish bowl

Salmon is known for its healthy omega-3 fats and is enjoyable served hot and cold, cooked or raw. A nourish bowl is very versatile as you can add many things to it. Our favourite is salmon (cooked and served how you please), a high-fibre carb like brown rice, loads of colourful veggies such as red cabbage, carrots, cucumber, sprouts, yellow capsicum and red onion, and then a serve of healthy fat like avocado, nuts or olive oil as a dressing. Don't forget to add some crunch with sesame seeds, dried chickpeas, or chopped nuts if you're more active.

Veggie-full lasagne

Lasagne is a fan favourite but try to use a little less pasta and meat and a little more vegetable throughout. We like to roast our veggies first then layer them into the lasagne. Ricotta is a nice, low-effort substitute for white sauce and if you can find some higher fibre pasta sheets, even better!

Curry with tofu, chickpeas and brown rice

Tofu is quite plain so needs to be served with other flavours that it can absorb. We like to marinate the tofu first or cook it in a curry loaded with vegetables. No tofu curry is complete without adding some legumes such as chickpeas and serving it over brown rice. There are some good curry spice blends/sauces on the market but be sure to read the ingredient labels to know what's really going into your meal. We also recommend using coconut milk over coconut cream for a lighter curry.

Let's talk about . . . alcohol and fat loss

Alcohol per gram is reasonably energy dense, and when metabolised produces close to 7 calories per gram of energy, which is almost as much as fat, at 9 calories.

The reality for a significant number of alcohol consumers is that they drink too much, too frequently, which has implications for both health and weight control.[93] What your alcohol is served with also impacts your health and weight-loss goals. Cocktails with juice or soft drink and spirits served with soft drink can add a lot of extra sugar and calories into the diet, which can make weight loss much harder. Cocktails also generally contain multiple shots of alcohol, which drive calories up even higher.

The link between alcohol and weight gain

It is commonly thought that alcohol causes weight gain as, per gram, alcohol is relatively high in calories. While alcohol does add to our caloric load, the weight gain we associate with drinking it is equally if not more attributable to the calorie-dense foods commonly served when enjoying a few drinks – think the fried food at the pub, the snack plate filled with cheese, salami and dips or the large plate of pasta you enjoy with a few glasses of red. The reason for this is that alcohol as a nutrient is metabolised before carbohydrates and fat, which means we are more likely to store the food calories that we consume when drinking alcohol at the same time.

Certainly, when fat loss is the goal, minimising your intake of alcohol is ideal as it otherwise adds extra calories into the diet. However, if you do want to include a glass of wine or a few drinks occasionally, the key is to be especially mindful of the calories you consume from food when you are drinking. Fried foods, pub-style food and snack platters are packed full of fat and calories, which means if you are also drinking alcohol more than occasionally, it will be difficult to achieve a calorie deficit that supports fat loss.

Is there a healthier alcohol?

Health-related content online frequently refers to the 'better' or 'healthier' alcohol options and while some drink varieties may be lower in calories, or have some antioxidants, ultimately there is no 'healthy' type of alcohol. Rather, whether your preference is for beer, wine or spirits, the best health message is to drink in moderation or, even better, not at all.

When you eat matters

When it comes to our general health and metabolism, meal timing and the mix of foods we eat at mealtimes matters. A simple focus on eating more calories earlier in the day and eating balanced meals and snacks will go a long way to ensuring your diet follows sound nutrition principles. Being mindful of what you eat and when is the foundation of a solid nutrition platform. But when it comes to healthy eating, nothing is as important as eating more vegetables, as you'll discover in the next chapter.

CHAPTER 9

VOLUME-EAT YOUR VEG

In this chapter we focus on packing your diet with nutrient-dense vegetables. Studies have shown that people who change their diet from a low-micronutrient diet to a high-micronutrient diet improve their experience of hunger. On a high-nutrient-density diet, hunger is not an unpleasant experience; rather, it is well tolerated and occurs with less frequency, even when meals are skipped (not that we're advocating that!).[94] So let's learn some easy ways to ensure your eating plan is packed full of foods with high micronutrient content.

Firstly, we'll teach you a core diet trick to transform your nutritional intake and power up your Burn phase: doubling your intake of vegetables and salad. This strategy, called volume eating, is a staple in the dietitians' toolkit.

While we are routinely told to aim for 5 vegetable serves and two fruit serves each day, this is really just the minimum required for health and wellbeing. In fact, for optimal health we should aim for at least 7 to 10 serves of low-calorie vegetables and fruits every single day.[95] When you are eating this much fresh food, not only are you getting the dietary fibre, antioxidants, vitamins and minerals you need for digestive health and glowing skin, but the large volume of fibrous food you are consuming helps to lower overall calorie intake and supports weight control.

Secondly, we'll share another brilliantly simple hack for those looking to manage their appetite and blood glucose: food sequencing.

Volume eating for fat loss

Volume eating is a concept that's been part of the dietitian's toolkit for quite some time, yet it has recently garnered attention in the media as a fresh approach to weight management. The strategy is straightforward: prioritise the consumption of high-volume, low-calorie foods such as fruits, vegetables, soups and whole grains, while moderating intake of calorie-dense items. This method allows for generous portions that satiate hunger without contributing excessive calories, thereby supporting weight-loss efforts.[96]

The roots of volume eating can be traced back to the work of nutrition scientist Barbara Rolls. This approach is grounded in the principle of consuming more nutrient-dense yet calorie-light foods, to create a sense of fullness and satisfaction. The high water and fibre content of these foods not only aids in maintaining a feeling of fullness but also contributes to overall digestive health.[97]

Volume eating offers several advantages. It promotes mindful eating, as the act of consuming fibre-rich foods requires more time and attention – literally, time spent chewing! – which in turn can lead to better recognition of satiety cues. Crucially, it's also a positive way to approach food, focusing on abundance rather than restriction, which can have beneficial psychological effects. With lots of beautiful, colourful produce on your plate, it's hard to feel deprived.

In essence, volume eating is a universally applicable method that aligns with healthful eating practices. It's an empowering way to enjoy a diversity of foods, support digestive health and manage weight effectively. It's an invitation to embrace the fullness of life, starting with what's on your plate.

Implementing volume eating in daily meals is not difficult, but it can take time to build the habit of including fresh food each and every time you eat. Taking a meal-by-meal approach is an easy way to start, by aiming for at least half to one cup of vegetables or salad as part of every meal or snack you eat.

For instance, a breakfast might include a bowl of oatmeal adorned with a variety of berries, a splash of low-fat milk with a sprinkle of protein powder. A lunch could be a substantial salad consisting of an assortment of roasted vegetables and starches, topped with a modest portion of protein. Dinner could involve a vibrant vegetable stir-fry accompanied by a lean source of protein and a small amount of high-fibre carbs. This approach ensures meals are visually appealing and nutritionally balanced. In doing this, you double or even triple the volume of food that's moving through your digestive system and likely decrease the overall calorie load compared to what you have previously been eating.

Volume-eating your veggies may be one of the easiest and most effective ways to stay on track with your weight-loss goals. By eating vegetables first and eating lots of them, you'll have less room for the higher calorie, lower nutrient foods that otherwise creep in. Don't be afraid to make your vegetables taste good, too! We'd rather you eat cauliflower with a little cheese on top or broccoli sauteed in garlic-infused olive oil than no vegetables at all.

Start at breakfast

While we do not always associate breakfast with vegetables, it is surprisingly easy to add them to the first meal of the day and thereby improve blood glucose control and fullness through the morning, thanks to the extra dietary fibre they contain. If you are an egg person, it's easy to add a side of tomatoes, mushrooms, baby spinach or onions. If cereal, muesli or porridge is your thing, you can easily grate in some extra zucchini, which blends straight in. Or if you prefer a liquid breakfast, you can always add a vegetable juice: a mix of greens, or beetroot, celery and carrot, blended and served with ice, offers a hit of antioxidants and dietary fibre (especially if you leave the skin on), for very few calories. If you are making a protein smoothie in the morning, try bulking it up with some extra cucumber, spinach leaves or kale.

Make lunch a meal

When we think of a meal versus a snack we grab on the run, one of the key differences is that a meal usually contains some salad or vegetables. On the other hand, quick lunches we pick up on the go, such as sushi, wraps or toasties, tend to contain very little salad or vegetable bulk – which is what we're looking to change. Swap those for veggie-full leftovers, a frozen meal, or consider adding an extra salad or soup to your regular lunch and get an extra 2 to 3 serves of fresh food in one sitting.

Add veg to any snacks

We are always keen to grab a protein or nut bar, or cheese and crackers when we feel like a snack, but we forget the importance of adding fresh food, such as a piece of fruit or vegetables, which add fibre bulk and extra nutrients to your day. Think fresh berries with yoghurt, cut-up vegetable sticks with a low-calorie dip like tzatziki, a vegetable juice or even a soup to go alongside any sweet, mid-morning or mid-afternoon snack.

Add a vegetable or salad course to your meals

We can learn a lot from different cultures when it comes to positive eating habits. The European habit of starting a meal with a light soup and ending it with some palate-cleansing leaves dressed in a little extra-virgin olive oil is not only a lovely mealtime ritual, but it will help you to eat fewer calories when the main meal is served, aid digestion and give you another 2 to 3 veggie serves at dinner. Studies have shown that you consume up to 100 fewer calories when you add a low-calorie vegetable course to any meal.[98] Even better is if you eat the vegetables or salad *first* – as we'll learn in food sequencing.

Get your plate balance right

Traditionally Aussies load their plates up with large serves of protein and plenty of starches via rice, potatoes and pasta, and if you are lucky there will also be a couple of spoons of coloured veggies added to the plate. Simply flipping these proportions so that veggies and salad fill half your plate, and your carbs and protein just a quarter each, will slash the calories of your meal by as much as half, while eating a similar volume of food overall. Utilising veggie-based rices and pastas, and making your vegetables taste great by roasting them, or adding them to dishes such as flavoursome pies, are easy ways to slip them into your favourite meals while significantly increasing that daily veg volume. We'll come back to this with plenty of examples in Chapter 10!

SUPERCHARGE YOUR FROZEN VEGETABLES

Cruciferous vegetables, which include broccoli, cauliflower, brussels sprouts and cabbage, are particularly well suited for freezing due to their robust structure and nutrient density. However, these veggies are prized for their health giving properties due to sulforaphane, a compound that can be deactivated during the freezing process. But don't worry, you can easily reactivate this powerful molecule with a little help from fresh foods rich in the necessary enzyme.[99]

When preparing your frozen vegetables, try adding a sprinkle of grated daikon radish or a dash of spicy mustard to the mix. These ingredients contain the enzyme myrosinase, which is needed to produce sulforaphane, reactivating the cancer-fighting potential of the vegetables. The amounts needed are minimal and won't alter the taste of your dish. Even after heating the veggies in the microwave, the reactivated compounds remain stable, ensuring you get the full spectrum of benefits.

By integrating this quick step into your cooking routine, you can turn your frozen vegetables into a supercharged, nutrient-packed component of your meals. It's an easy, affordable way to enhance the nutritional value of convenient frozen veggies, helping you and your family enjoy a healthful diet without compromising on the powerful anti-cancer properties these foods can offer.

Meet Kara: over-hungry and eating off the kids' plates 🛒

At 42, Kara was the epitome of an exhausted mum, juggling the never-ending demands of parenthood with a full-time job. Her goals were straightforward yet elusive: to chip away at her stubborn 'mum tum' by losing 5 to 10 kilograms, curb the mindless munching and find a way to boost her energy levels.

Kara had a mixed bag of dietary habits. While her meals were fairly healthy, they lacked balance, with too many carbs at dinner and not enough protein at breakfast. She didn't eat afternoon tea, a well-intentioned sacrifice in the pursuit of weight loss that only left her ravenous by evening, leading to her nibbling off her children's dinner plates. Weekends were a snacking spree, often beginning with a skipped breakfast and ending with hunger pangs that led to impulsive eating.

A key challenge hinged on Kara's lunches, which were too light and lacking in substance – often just boiled eggs on crackers, or a tuna salad. She needed more bulk in the form of protein, veggies and wholegrain carbs in the middle of the day. After such a light lunch, the convenience of her children's eye-level snacks was a siren call she struggled to resist later in the day. Meal planning was a foreign concept in the hectic flow of her life and, with constant fatigue weighing her down, it usually felt easier to just bend to her kids' unhealthy dinner requests.

With help from her dietitian, the turnaround began with a family huddle and a whiteboard on the fridge, mapping out the week's lunches and dinners and simplifying the grocery shopping. To ensure a steady supply of fresh, healthy options the new routine became two shopping trips per week – one of them delivered to home for ease.

Kara's husband, recognising her weariness, offered to cook twice a week, and they decided to use healthy frozen meals with an extra portion of frozen veggies as a reprieve on Thursdays and Fridays, their most tiring evenings. As a family, they also committed to always having some extra serves of vegetables or salads in the middle of the table so anyone could add extra bulk to their meal if they wished. Kara swapped her light lunches for more volume-filling leftover portions from dinner, which were also more satisfying, particularly in the winter months.

Kara armed herself for weekend sports with overnight oats or chia pudding loaded up with mixed berries, a strategic move to fend off post-game snack attacks. She banished the children's snacks to a lidded box at the bottom of the pantry where they'd be safely out of sight and mind, and instead had mason jars in the fridge filled with water and chopped veggie sticks (so they remained fresh and crunchy all week long), which became an easy snack to grab with some dip or salsa. And in the evenings while her kids ate their dinner, Kara would journal, focusing on her goals instead of the food on their plates.

Twelve weeks after implementing these changes, Kara was 6.8 kilograms lighter, feeling a new, steadier level of energy and no longer subject to the dreaded afternoon slump. She slipped into old clothes with renewed confidence and was able to exercise control over her food choices, both at home and at work. Meal planning became intentional, her eating driven by hunger rather than habit – a victory for the once-weary mum who had found her stride.

NOTES FROM THE NUTRITION COUCH
HOW GUT HEALTH RELATES TO FAT LOSS AND OBESITY

Research from Nottingham Trent University suggests our gut has more to do with weight gain than you might think, due to microbe fragments called endotoxins that can enter the bloodstream and impact the function of fat cells. In a nutshell, it means poor gut health may impact our ability to lose weight.[100]

While it may seem like an easy fix, improving gut health isn't as simple as grabbing some probiotics from the chemist or cutting out gluten. Instead, view gut health as an ongoing process of maintenance. We know that consuming a high number (30 or more) of plant-based, fibre-filled foods each week can be one of the most powerful things you can do for good gut health.

So, as a first step concentrate on your day-to-day food choices and keep consistent with a healthy diet.

13 August 2023[101]

Food sequencing

Food sequencing is the tactic of eating your vegetables first, then protein and fats, before finishing with carbohydrates, which can be a powerful way to keep blood glucose levels controlled and support you in feeling fuller and more satisfied after eating.

It has also been shown to help improve one's overall nutrient intake as it prioritises healthier foods – more fruits, vegetables and lean protein and fewer heavy carbohydrates – and to reduce the risk of cardiovascular disease, cancer and and all-cause mortality.[102]

It is suggested that food sequencing may help reduce and prevent the glucose highs and lows that can be experienced by individuals with blood-glucose–regulation issues including hypoglycaemia, insulin resistance or pre- or type 2 diabetes.[103] As each of the macronutrients – carbohydrate, protein and fat – are digested at different rates, studies have found that front-loading a meal with high-fibre, protein and higher fat foods before eating carbohydrates can help keep blood-glucose levels more tightly regulated. Ingestion of lipids (fats) and protein before carbo-hydrate, as a 'preload', has been shown to acutely improve glucose tolerance, mainly by delaying gastric emptying and enhancing insulin secretion.[104]

Additionally, it helps to promote feelings of satiety thereby reducing overall calorie intake.[105] Studies in the area of volumet-rics, where a low-calorie, fibre-rich salad, soup or vegetable-based dish is consumed before a meal, have shown that subsequent calorie intake is significantly reduced. It is thought that the fibre and bulk of such a vegetable preload helps to slow digestion and manage appetite, partly due to promoting the secretion of peptide GLP-1, which plays a key role in regulating insulin in the body and helping to delay gastric emptying, which in turn supports glucose regulation.[106] Moreover, eating fruits, vegetables and lean proteins first tends to prioritise them in the diet, rebalancing nutrient intake to favour a healthier eating pattern.[107]

How do you 'food sequence'?

While the science of food sequencing is still emerging, it could be useful to try if you struggle with cravings, constant hunger and/or glucose highs and lows. The good news is that it is rela-tively easy to implement. In essence, you're not changing what you eat as much as the order in which you eat it. If you are already eating balanced meals, this theory suggests that simply by changing the sequence of consumption, you may dial up their benefits further.

In practice, food sequencing looks like eating low-energy-density foods like salads or soups first, followed by protein-rich foods such as chicken, meat or dairy, and ending the meal with starchy carbohydrates. Simply start any meal with a high-fibre, low-calorie food. For example, a bowl of berries before your breakfast meal, or a soup, salad or veggies at the start of lunch or dinner. Follow this with a protein, such as eggs, meat, chicken, fish, tofu or legumes, before finishing with a serve of wholefood carbohydrate.

One of the advantages of food sequencing is that it prioritises choosing good quality and correctly portioned carbohydrates. For instance, eating this way would encourage you to eat a whole jacket potato instead of mashed potato (which combines the carbohydrate with fats, and thus should be eaten separately). Such choices align with dietary recommendations for carbohydrate quality. In addition, because each meal starts with fruits or vegetables these are prioritised in the diet, which is beneficial for weight loss and delivers many positive health outcomes.

The approach is a novel one. While it might not be universally necessary, those with blood-sugar concerns may find it a useful tool for metabolic benefits and in managing glucose control. In addition, you may feel more satisfied and have fewer cravings, thanks to slower gastric emptying.

Veggies are your secret weapon

Whether your goal is to feel better, lose weight, improve your digestion or hormones, or have more energy, the simplest, most effective thing you can focus on from a diet perspective is to eat more vegetables. Whether you enjoy your vegetables cooked, raw, juiced or blended, considering less than 10 per cent of Australians eat the recommended amount of vegetables each day, chances are you too will benefit from eating more. So, start by making sure each of your meals and snacks contains some fresh food, and notice how much better you start to feel very quickly.

CHAPTER 10

FOLLOW OUR FAT-LOSS FORMULA

It feels like there are a million different diets out there, all with different calorie and carbohydrate loads and all claiming to hold the answer to weight loss. You can become consumed with counting calories, or carbohydrate or fat grams, and no matter which diet it is, chances are you end up right back where you started. Why? Because such a strict approach is generally unsustainable long term.

We do have good news, though! The secret to fat loss is not any strict regime that requires weighing foods or counting calories, but instead a very simple formula that will turn your healthy eating into sustainable results.

You see, it's all to do with portion control and the correct macronutrient distribution. If you remember to balance every one of your meals with a serve of good quality carbohydrates, a serve of lean protein, a serve of good fat and 3 serves of vegetables or salads, you can solve a great deal of common dietary issues and shed some unwanted body fat along the way. It is this mix that helps to regulate appetite by ensuring you have a meal that will keep you feeling full and satisfied for several hours, while also keeping blood-glucose levels stable and cravings at bay.

Healthy eating versus eating for fat loss

In this book and in our clinical practices, we will always prioritise health over fat loss because your long-term overall health is the most important thing and we never want our clients to chase fat loss at the expense of their health. Health must be the first priority as if you're eating a lot of ultra-processed foods, takeaways and alcohol, even if you are losing body fat, this way of eating isn't good for your long-term health.

However, while making healthy eating choices is the priority, eating healthy doesn't automatically equate to fat loss. And in order to look after your health long term, maintaining a healthy weight is vital. The challenge is real. You can be eating very healthily and filling your body with plenty of nourishing wholefoods, but if you're eating too much of these good foods, you'll struggle to lose body fat. Yes, you read that correctly, you can fuel your body by eating lots of nourishing foods but if you are not in a calorie deficit, that will not translate to fat loss.

To achieve a calorie deficit, you need to eat fewer calories than the body requires. Assuming there are no other factors that may be impacting your weight, if your weight is stable, you are eating at maintenance. If your weight is increasing, you are eating in a calorie surplus (more than your body needs). And if your weight is decreasing (that is, you are achieving fat loss), you are eating less than your body currently needs.

It might seem counterintuitive, from a health perspective, to actively eat less than your body requires. But if you are aiming to lose 10 kilograms, as an example, you need to 'eat down' to create that body. If you want to inhabit a body that weighs 10 kilograms less than the body you are in now, you need to eat the amount of food that will sustain your new, smaller body. Put simply, you need to eat less.

CALORIE TARGETS FOR FAT LOSS

Calories matter for fat loss as you actively need to be in a calorie deficit to lose weight. Eating less than your body requires is difficult to predict as we are all individuals. Calorie targets can differ depending on your gender, age, height, weight, muscle mass, activity levels, clinical conditions and background.

In order to determine your current daily calorie requirement, the simplest approach, as discussed in the Nourish for Energy chapter, is to determine your basal metabolic rate and add this to any extra energy demands to account for your activity levels and additional needs. There are numerous online calculators available to help you, but be warned, they often overestimate requirements (as they're mostly based on young male subjects who have more muscle mass) so take them with a grain of salt and adjust as needed. Also remember, to work towards weight loss you will need to lower your maintenance calories by around 300 to 500 calories a day. Ideally, though, it's best to work with a health practitioner to get these numbers accurate for you and continue to adjust your plan over time so you continue to lose fat.

Below is a rough guide for the average 30- to 50-year-old female wanting to lose 10 to 20 kilograms, to achieve consistent, sustainable fat loss. However, you will need to work out your own targets based on your body and lifestyle, taking into account the factors outlined above.

MEAL	ESTIMATED CALORIE TARGETS
Breakfast	300 to 400 calories
Lunch	400 to 500 calories
Dinner	400 to 500 calories
Snacks/drinks/treats	200 to 400 calories
Daily total range =	1300 to 1800 calories

Food labels

Knowledge is power, particularly when trying to achieve a calorie deficit. Understanding how much energy is in the foods you choose can be the difference between losing weight and staying the same. Just because you order a salad, it doesn't automatically mean that it will meet your goals of fat loss – the ingredients and the portion size matter. This is where reading food labels and understanding the energy density of foods is very helpful. You want to choose foods that have healthy ingredients on the labels (or better still, no labels at all – hello, fresh fruit!) and choose products that have lower energy or calories per serve compared to other products in the range. Achieving health and fat loss is a delicate balance between both the ingredients and overall energy in the products/foods.

Let us break this down for you. As an example, if your current lunch is a large full-cream milk coffee and a large muffin from a café and you swapped that to a chicken and quinoa pesto salad, while this may be a better choice nutritionally, the calories are probably similar, so it's unlikely to support fat loss. Even though it may be a healthier option due to the addition of more macro- and micronutrients (protein, salads, fibre, et cetera) and you may get some down-the-line benefits of feeling fuller for longer, on balance, your calorie intake remains the same.

If instead you chose a small chicken wrap with a big garden salad on the side, this is also a healthier choice but, importantly for weight loss, the difference is that it's a less energy-dense option thanks to the bulk of the meal coming from a low-calorie, nutrient-rich salad, while the protein and carbohydrate portions are smaller. This macro adjustment, which volumises fibre and all its health benefits as previously outlined, should contribute to fat loss – providing the rest of your day also runs at a calorie deficit.

A good way to understand the difference between eating healthy and eating for fat loss is to compare healthy meals with their equivalents that come in at around 300 to 400 calories. It's important to note that both options in the table are healthy and nourishing, but one supports fat loss while the other supports weight maintenance.

EXAMPLES OF HEALTHY MEALS THAT TARGET WEIGHT MAINTENANCE (AROUND 400 CALORIES)	EXAMPLES OF HEALTHY MEALS THAT TARGET FAT LOSS (AROUND 300 CALORIES)
Homemade Beef Burgers Making your own beef patties to stack between a hamburger bun is a great option instead of takeaway. Adding cheese, salad and a little mayo/relish are all good options for a nourishing meal. Depending on your hunger/activity levels, a serve of oven-baked chips may be added.	**Naked Burgers and Salad** Extra-lean beef burger patties that you can find at most supermarkets contain around 100 calories per serve, which means you can enjoy 2 to 3 naked burger patties (without a bun) with plenty of salad for a light yet satisfying meal. You can also make your own using premium beef mince and adding grated veggies.
Beef Stir-fry with Noodles A high-protein and high-iron option, lean beef strips can be a great addition to the family stir-fry. Adding noodles and vegetables plus a lower sugar/salt sauce can keep the whole family happy while ensuring you are putting some great nutrients into your body.	**Prawn Stir-fry** Prawns are often overlooked for both their protein and low calorie content. A large portion (200 grams) of raw prawns contains fewer than 200 calories. This means you can enjoy a prawn stir-fry with a little soy sauce, veggies and cauliflower rice or konjac noodles for a low-carb, low-calorie meal.
Beef Meatballs and Pasta Using beef mince to make your own meatballs is a great, nourishing choice. Grating in some veggies is also a good idea to boost the nutrients. Choosing a high-fibre pasta and adding some cheese on top is a great way to round out the meal and adds beneficial calcium and carbohydrates.	**Turkey/Chicken Meatballs** A lean, high-protein meat, turkey can be made into a tasty meatball or spaghetti sauce with zucchini noodles and extra vegetables, which in total clocks in at a very lean 300 calories.

EXAMPLES OF HEALTHY MEALS THAT TARGET WEIGHT MAINTENANCE (AROUND 400 CALORIES)	EXAMPLES OF HEALTHY MEALS THAT TARGET FAT LOSS (AROUND 300 CALORIES)
Crumbed Fish, Chips and Salad A homemade variety of this is far better from a health perspective than takeaway fish and chips. Use wholemeal crumbs on the fish, extra-virgin olive oil on your potato and pop them in to bake in the oven or air-fryer instead of deep-frying them. Ensure you add some salad to the plate for a nourishing meal.	**Grilled Fish and Roasted Vegetables** While tuna and salmon are on the higher calorie side thanks to their rich omega-3 content, if you stick to white fish and pair it with a bucket-load of lower carb veggies such as zucchini, eggplant, capsicum, onion and pumpkin, you will strike a perfect balance for a lighter fat-burning dinner.
Vegetable Quiche A homemade version using lots of vegetables, eggs and a light pastry will mean that this is a far better choice than a shop-bought one, which often has added cream, bacon and full-fat pastry.	**Veggie Frittata** Who said that eggs should be limited to breakfast? In fact, a crustless frittata made with eggs, lots of grated vegetables and a little cheese equates to 250 to 300 calories in a relatively large slice and can be enjoyed with salad for a filling, nutrient-rich lunch or dinner meal.
Salmon Cakes with Wedges and Salad Using tinned salmon to make patties can be an easy and nourishing dinner option. The whole family can enjoy the patties with added cheese, grated veggies, breadcrumbs and eggs. Pan-fry them in some extra-virgin olive oil and add some oven-baked wedges and salad to the plate.	**Salmon Cakes and Salad** While a large piece of fresh salmon can bump up your calorie intake, mixing a small can of tinned salmon with some cottage cheese, grated vegetables, eggs and a light seasoning of breadcrumbs keeps the carbs and calories low for a great-tasting, quick and easy dinner. Don't forget to load up your plate with lots of fresh and colourful salad.

EXAMPLES OF HEALTHY MEALS THAT TARGET WEIGHT MAINTENANCE (AROUND 400 CALORIES)	EXAMPLES OF HEALTHY MEALS THAT TARGET FAT LOSS (AROUND 300 CALORIES)
BBQ Chicken Wraps and Salad This is a quick and easy meal option you can grab from the supermarket on your way home. Just ensure your wraps are higher fibre, add some fats (like avocado) on the wrap, too, for satiety and include a side salad.	**BBQ Chicken and Salad** A family favourite for a quick weeknight lunch or dinner. Just remember to take the skin off the chicken and pass on the stuffing and chips, all of which are high in fat. Stick to lean chicken breast, a serve of healthy fats like avocado or olives, and load up on your favourite salads to build a balanced and fat-burning meal.
Sushi Keep your choices focused on brown rice sushi rolls and leaner proteins like chicken breast, salmon and tuna. Adding some edamame can also boost the protein and fibre. Go easy on any deep-fried and mayonnaise-loaded options.	**Sashimi, Edamame and Seaweed Salad** If the rest of the family is getting takeaway sushi, this option is the perfect way for you to order in, too, but still keep the meal light and higher-protein for satiety. The edamame and seaweed salad provide some carbs and fibre for fullness and the sashimi provides healthy fats and protein to help support your metabolism. If salt isn't a concern for you, add a miso soup.
Minestrone Soup and Wholegrain Toast There's nothing better than minestrone soup in winter with some wholegrain toast and a light spread of butter. It's an easy and nutritious way to get in loads of fibre, nutrients and slower digesting carbs.	**Vegetable and Legume Soup** There's nothing better than a hearty bowl of vegetable soup for fat loss but be sure to add some beans or legumes such as kidney beans or chickpeas for extra protein, fibre and fullness. No need to add toast to your portion as the beans provide some carbs for fuel.

EXAMPLES OF HEALTHY MEALS THAT TARGET WEIGHT MAINTENANCE (AROUND 400 CALORIES)	EXAMPLES OF HEALTHY MEALS THAT TARGET FAT LOSS (AROUND 300 CALORIES)
Beef Kebabs and Grilled Corn with Flatbread An easy summer dinner that is high in protein and provides a good mix of carbs for fuel, protein for satiety and veggies for fullness.	**Marinated Tofu and Vegetable Kebabs** There is a growing range of marinated tofu or tempeh in the supermarket that can make for a quick and easy plant-based protein source for dinner. Simply cut into pieces and thread onto skewers, alternating with as many different coloured vegetables as possible. Cook kebabs on your barbecue grill plate and add some salsa or sriracha as a lower calorie dressing option if needed. Add some grilled corn as a side if you're hungry, active or need a calorie boost.

As you can see, with some smart and simple swaps, you can take your meals from maintenance phase to fat-burn phase during periods in life when you want or need to manage your weight more closely, while knowing you'll still be well nourished.

Meet Christa: the difference between healthy eating and eating for fat loss

Christa was 46, a picture of health on the surface, and yet the results she sought – shedding body fat and trimming her waistline – proved stubbornly difficult to reach. She was the epitome of someone who ate well and stayed active but didn't see the changes she hoped for.

Her diet was commendable overall, rich in organic foods, with minimal takeaway and no alcohol. But it was not a dietary pattern tailored for fat loss. Christa's daily routine included two full-cream milk coffees and the occasional weekend treat of an organic acai bowl. Generous handfuls of trail mix consisting of nuts, seeds and dried fruit was her go-to snack, and she enjoyed rich meals that often featured multiple serves of healthy fats: cheese, olives, avocado, hemp seeds, dukkah and olive oil–based dressings. She'd eat 4 or 5 large salmon fillets each week as she knew that the healthy fats in salmon were key for anti-inflammatory eating.

Christa's Greek heritage meant that flavourful, fat-rich meals were a cultural staple, but her portions – especially the trail mix and salmon – were more than her body needed for fat loss. The challenge was clear: her calorie intake was simply too high to allow her body to burn fat.

The solution was multifaceted. Christa invested in non-stick pans to cut down on the generous olive oil pour she used to cook every meal and she started portioning out her trail mix to avoid over-indulgence. Dried fruit as a snack was swapped for fresh fruit, and her full-cream milk was replaced with a lighter alternative. She cut down on salmon meals and added variety to her diet with other proteins like fish, lean pork, chicken, tofu and legumes. To boost her muscle mass and metabolism, she began doing strength training with a personal trainer twice a week and made a habit of walking after dinner on her home treadmill.

The results spoke volumes. Christa's waistline shrank from 86 centimetres down to 80 centimetres, and she dropped two dress sizes. Her cholesterol levels improved, earning her doctor's praise. With a better grip on nutrition tailored for fat loss, she felt her confidence in her clothes improving after only a few months. Perhaps most importantly, her approach to meals became more mindful, leaving her feeling content and in control after eating. Christa's journey was a testament to the power of nuanced changes, proving that healthy eating and eating for fat loss, while seemingly similar, require different strategies and attention to detail.

Our fat-burning meal formula

It is commonly recommended that healthy adults wanting to lose weight aim to achieve a 15 to 20 per cent calorie reduction from their current requirements each day. Practically, this translates to around a 250 to 400 calorie deficit most days depending on how overweight you are to start with and how much you're aiming to lose. As outlined in the boxed guidelines above, each person's needs are different, so this can only be a rough guide.

Some determine their deficit by tracking or counting their calories and macros, which can be very time consuming and may even promote disordered eating in some people. Others significantly increase the amount of exercise they do, which in our experience is a challenge to maintain long term and tends to increase your hunger, making consistent fat loss harder as time goes on. And others still work with a dietitian who may calculate this for them – but this isn't financially or practically accessible for everyone.

Our alternative is a simple formula that helps the majority of our clients achieve a calorie deficit and promote fat loss. With that said, everyone is an individual so you may want to get some personalised advice from a dietitian if you have any medical conditions or unusual requirements.

This fat-loss meal formula is something we have both used ourselves, particularly to shed the postpartum baby weight. We also recommend it to our family and friends who are trying to lose stubborn weight. It works well for our clients as they find they are able to use it at home, adapting it for the whole family, but also in social situations and on holidays. It's something that takes some time and practice but, once implemented regularly, becomes second nature and makes losing and maintaining the weight easier in the long term.

The formula is a huge bonus in your toolkit as it isn't about restriction, but about choice and volume eating. Rather than a strict set of rules or foods you can and can't eat, you get to choose what goes on your plate based on how you're feeling each day. No foods are off limits, but you do need to make a conscious choice at each mealtime to ensure you're only choosing one option from each macronutrient so the formula works. Fat loss doesn't have to be bland, boring, repetitive or restrictive – it can be nourishing, tasty, flavoursome, volume-based and filled with the foods you and your family enjoy.

The bottom line is, if the goal is fat loss you need to ensure your overall energy balance for the day is in a mild to moderate deficit. Ultimately, calories are the key, so finding the right balance is important. However, our fat-loss formula should naturally reduce the calories of your meals and can be a useful, general approach without calorie counting. That said, if you are in a body that is unusually small or large, or active, it may help to see a dietitian who can help you calculate your calorie requirements and advise meal choices that will best help you hit the right numbers for your fat-loss goal.

The fat-burning meal formula for a small or average female

Often in our quest for fat loss we make things complicated – we cut out the carbs, we increase the protein too much or we overdo the good fats. But the secret is simple: fill your plates in the proportions illustrated on the following page and this will naturally help create a calorie deficit while still leaving you with plenty of food at regular mealtimes, without the need to eliminate food groups or go hungry.

This is straightforward enough, but until people have learnt and practised the formula they will often imbalance the ratios. It can be easy to overdo the carbs, fats and protein but miss out on the necessary fresh produce, which is why having a formula to remind you of the ratios is really handy. It's also important to note that you should be aiming for lean proteins, and mostly plant-based healthy fats.

Carbs: 1 serve
For example:
- ½ cup cooked pasta or
  rice
- 1 medium baked potato
- small bread roll
- cob of corn

**Fibre – salad/veggies:
3 serves**
For example:
1 serve = 1 cup salad or
½ cup cooked veggies
(fruit in small amounts,
see below)

On a plate these
serving sizes
will look roughly
like this.

Protein: 1 serve
For example:
- palm-sized piece of lean
  protein such as chicken,
  steak, tofu or fish
- 2 eggs
- ¾ cup of beans

Fat: 1 serve
For example:
- 1 tbsp oil, nut butter,
  mayo or pesto
- 30 g cheese
- 25 g nuts
- ¼ avocado

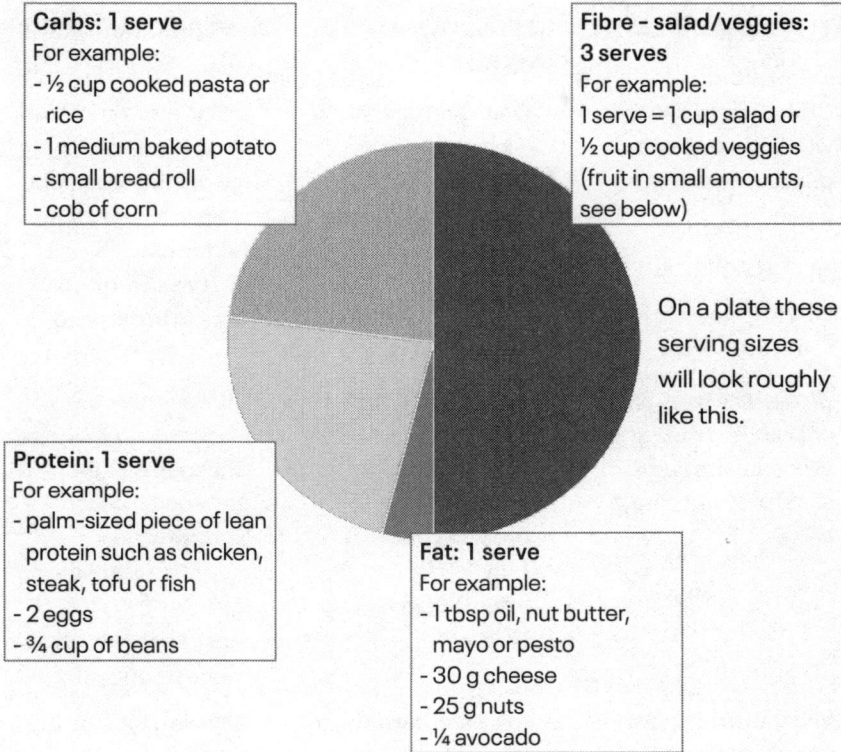

While it's important to meet your daily calcium and vitamin D requirements, especially for women as we age, if your goal is fat loss, try to limit too much full-fat dairy and count it towards the fat targets above. Be aware, too, that plant-based milks can contain a lot of sugar, which will add to your calorie intake. If you do choose to use them, stick to ones with no or low sugar and ensure they are calcium-fortified.

We haven't included fruits in the above portions, as they should be enjoyed in low amounts while pursuing fat-loss goals. One or two serves a day of fruit (ideally with the skin on) can fit into a balanced eating plan but just be aware of your overall energy intake if your goal is to lose body fat.

Let's apply our formula to some favourite meals to show how they can still be enjoyed while supporting fat loss.

TYPICAL MEAL EATEN	BREAKDOWN OF MACROS	SIMPLE 'FORMULA' FIX
Crumbed chicken tacos with lettuce, cheese, guacamole and sour cream	• Crumbing on chicken + in taco shells = 2 carbs • Cheese, guacamole and sour cream = 3 fats • Chicken = 1 protein • Lettuce = 1 veg	• Grilled chicken instead • Choose one of the following: guacamole, cheese or sour cream • Add an extra 2 cups of extra salad to your plate to boost veggies
Burger with beef, bacon, cheese, lettuce, tomato, avocado, aioli and a serve of sweet potato chips	• Burger bun + chips = 2 carbs • Beef and bacon = 2 protein • Avocado, aioli and fried chips = 3 fats • Lettuce/tomato slice = 1 veg	• Choose either the burger bun or the chips • Choose either the beef patty or the bacon • Choose either avocado, aioli or the fries • Add a huge side salad to boost veggies
Vegetarian big breakfast with eggs, baked beans, half a tomato, sourdough toast, halloumi, avocado and pesto	• Toast and baked beans = 2 carbs • Halloumi, pesto and avocado = 3 fats • Eggs = 1 protein • ½ tomato = ½ veg	• Choose either toast or baked beans • Choose either halloumi, pesto or avocado • Add extra veggies
Tomato pasta with olive oil and garlic bread	• 2 cups of pasta + piece of garlic bread = 5 serves of carbs • Tomato in pasta = 1 veg • Minimal protein • Oil to cook and drizzled on pasta = 1 fat	• Reduce pasta amount to half a cup and remove garlic bread • Add protein to the pasta, e.g. chicken • Add extra veggies or a big side salad
Tuna salad with a whole avocado, cucumber and mixed leaves	• Tuna = 1 protein • Avocado = 4 fats • Cucumber and mixed leaves = 2 veg • No carb portion	• Add in a carb serve, e.g. roasted potato • Reduce avocado to ¼ • Add in 1–2 more veggie serves

How 'go light at night' fits into our fat-burning meal formula

If you have a hormonal condition such as PCOS, insulin resistance or are in the peri-menopause years, you may want to consider reducing your calorie and carbohydrate load at night.[108] In this case, adjust our fat-loss formula by reducing or removing the carbohydrate portion at your dinner meal to assist with further fat burning. You may choose to do this a few days of the week or on the majority of days, based on the results you are getting.

Flexibility with the formula is key

As we know, nothing in life is perfect. Sometimes we overeat despite our best intentions, so we wanted to remind you that this journey isn't about perfection, but about consistency and flexibility. If you have a larger or more calorie-dense meal, feel free to adapt the fat-loss formula based on what your hunger is telling you. If for example, you have a large 3-course lunch and you're not that hungry come dinner time, you may want to just have a light chicken salad or a veggie and bean soup for dinner instead (and lose the carb and fat portions). We don't recommend regularly missing key macro- or micronutrients from this formula, but on the odd occasion you may over-indulge, adjusting the formula is perfectly okay.

It is also fine to adjust it based on a recipe's ingredients or taste profile. Say, for example, you wanted to make a salad with a beautiful creamy dressing that included cheese but had no carbs. Rather than adding the carb into the recipe as it was never there to begin with, you keep the double fat portion in the recipe, allowing it to replace the carb portion. Just remember, it's important to apply these adjustments at your discretion. Overall, we recommend most meals match our fat-loss meal formula as it's easy, filling and supportive of fat loss.

Top breakfasts to support fat loss

A well-balanced breakfast that supports calorie control and fat loss will contain 20 grams of protein and 20 to 40 grams of carbohydrate per serve. We appreciate that adding veggies into breakfast is not always possible, so try to focus on fibre with breakfast and include a serve of fresh fruit if you're not adding vegetables.

Eggs on toast

When it comes to the best breakfast meals for fat loss, it is tough to go past eggs. With 14 grams of high quality protein per serve of 2 large eggs, along with 11 other vitamins and minerals, they make the perfect addition to your breakfast. Team them with some wholegrain toast (carbs) and veggies cooked in olive oil (fat) and garlic to complete your fat-burning meal and align it with our formula.

Breakfast cereal

If cereal is your breakfast preference, the key to achieving the right mix of carbs and protein is to make your favourite cereal into a protein- and fibre-rich breakfast bowl by adding high-protein yoghurt or protein powder. Simply team one-third to half a cup of oats, or your favourite wholegrain cereal (carbs), with high-protein Greek yoghurt or 2 tablespoons of protein powder (protein), a little chopped fruit (fibre) and a tablespoon of seeds or nuts (fats) and let it set in the fridge overnight. The simple addition of fibre and protein makes this breakfast exceptionally filling and delicious.

Protein toast

With a growing range of higher protein bread options available in supermarkets, you are now able to enjoy your favourite spreads with a good toast. These breads are high in protein, fat and fibre but are typically low in carbohydrates, so try to add some carbs on your toast to follow the fat-burning meal formula. A full meal includes 1 to 2 slices of low-carb, high-protein toast with some banana, honey and cinnamon; or ricotta, honey and strawberries. This is a nice balanced breakfast supportive of your fat-loss goals.

Breakfast wrap

If you need convenient breakfast options that you can grab on the go, do not forget that your favourite lunch wrap can be quickly turned into a high-protein brekky option. Smoked salmon (protein) with cream cheese (fat) and salad (fibre) is the perfect breakfast wrap filling. If you're not a fan of smoked salmon, try turkey (protein) with avocado (fat) and some cucumber (fibre); or for a vegetarian protein boost, pair black beans (protein) with goat's cheese (fat), salsa and some tomatoes (fibre).

Protein smoothies

Another grab-and-go option that can be prepared in advance is blending Greek yoghurt (protein) with your choice of milk, fruit (carbs) and nuts or seeds (fats) to make a smoothie that would easily reach 15 to 20 grams of protein. Or if you prefer to use protein powder, simply add 2 tablespoons of your favourite protein powder (protein) with fresh fruit (carbs), nut butter (fat) and ice or milk and this will create a filling breakfast smoothie with 20 to 30 grams of protein per serve.

Top lunches to support fat loss

A well-balanced lunch that includes 100 to 150 grams of lean protein such as meat, chicken or fish with 1 to 2 serves of good quality carbohydrates, a portion of healthy fats and 2 to 3 cups of salad or vegetables will keep you full and satisfied throughout the afternoon, with fewer cravings and less desire to snack. Quick options such as sushi, dumplings or sandwiches tend to lack the bulk of a large salad or side of vegetables with your lunch, and once you add this component back in you will notice how much more in control of your appetite and energy you are throughout the afternoon.

Soup or salad with a sandwich

When we are wanting to achieve a calorie deficit, our default can be to start too strict, and keep lunch overly light with a plain tuna salad or sushi roll. The issue with this is that while salad is a good choice, unless it contains a decent portion of protein and good quality carbohydrate, you will be hungry again an hour or two later. A much better option is a salad or soup (for the veggie bulk) as well as a small sandwich or wrap that includes some protein like chicken or tuna and healthy fats like avocado or cheese. Not only will the vegetable bulk in the soup help to keep you full but the serve of carbs and protein in the sandwich or wrap will keep you satisfied for several hours.

A substantial salad

We are not talking about a few leaves and a tin of tuna here, but rather 2 to 3 cups of salad ingredients along with a palm-sized portion of protein such as chicken breast, lean lamb, salmon or a couple of eggs and a decent serve of carbs via a slice of wholegrain bread, or half cup of brown rice, sweet potato or beans. Most importantly, a serve of good fat from some olive oil dressing or a quarter of a small avocado will help to keep you full for several hours. Remember that you are always better off making your own salad as food court options tend to be packed with extra fats and calories coming from cheese, nuts, heavy carb portions like rice or pasta, and lashings of dressing.

Leftovers

The beauty with leftovers is that they are not only cost-effective but also allow you to control your calorie intake. As it is lunch you can also include a decent serve of carbs via rice, pasta or potato without impacting your weight-loss attempts. You may have also noticed that enjoying a hot meal at lunch is much more satisfying than a comparatively unappealing salad or sandwich that you have been used to grabbing for years, if not decades. Good examples include a chicken and cashew stir-fry served with brown rice, a high-fibre pasta salad with tuna, feta and extra veggies, or mini frittatas served with a slice of toast and a side salad with olive oil dressing.

A frozen or pre-made meal

There is a growing range of calorie-controlled, nutritious frozen and pre-made meal options available at supermarkets that contain just 300 to 500 calories per serve, which can be a perfect quick, easy and convenient lunch option, and one that also keeps your calorie intake controlled. Try to seek out options that contain 20 to 30 grams of protein per serve, 40 grams of carbs or less and a few serves of vegetables, as this will align well with your fat-burning meal formula.

Top dinners to support fat loss

A meal that includes a serve of just 100 to 150 grams of cooked lean protein, a portion of healthy fats, 2 to 3 cups of salad or vegetables and a portion-controlled, half-cup serve of carbs such as brown rice or wholemeal pasta, if needed, will give you around 400 calories or less in a meal that supports sustainable fat loss.

SIMPLE DINNERS THAT FOCUS ON FLAVOUR AND FULLNESS

- Stir-fries with cauliflower rice (e.g. prawns cooked in olive oil with 2 to 3 cups of veggies and cauli rice).
- Lean meatballs with zucchini noodles (serve with parmesan cheese for flavour, counted in your fats, and include some wholemeal breadcrumbs in the meatballs if you're wanting some carbs).
- Grilled fish or chicken with roasted vegetables (add pesto to your protein for some healthy fats and ensure you include some roasted potato or sweet potato if you're wanting the carb portion).

- Naked beef burrito bowl with salad (adding black beans can provide carbs, and avocado or cheese is a tasty way to include some fats in the meal).
- Roasted vegetable salad with pork (quinoa can provide some high-fibre carbs if needed, and a nice olive oil, mustard and red wine vinegar dressing can add flavour; don't forget to add some baby spinach leaves to the roasted veggies to increase the volume).
- Bowl of soup (add chickpeas for protein, a little brown rice for carbs, if wanted, and serve with a sprinkle of cheese for flavour, counted in your fats).
- Vegetable omelette (cheese works well as a fat serve and adding some extra egg whites gives a good protein boost; if wanting to add carbs, include 1 to 2 slices of grainy toast).
- Tuna or salmon patties with salad (add some breadcrumbs to the patties for carbs, and some nuts or seeds in the salad to provide some healthy fats and extra fibre).

Our 10 structured steps for weight loss

So now you know what eating for fat loss looks like and you have a handy formula that's ready to go. Before we close this final chapter, we want to recap some key pieces of wisdom to help you keep powering along in fat-burning mode.

While a strict plan to stick to can help with short-term weight loss, often the smallest slip off the plan can mean you're totally off the rails and the diet is done. Instead, we recommend some structure with your nutrition – not rigid food rules but 10 key steps that will keep you on track in a much more sustainable way. Yes, they all require some commitment! But these simple yet powerful dietary changes offer numerous benefits for your long-term weight, health and wellbeing, so it's worth it. If you commit long term to this new way of eating and living, you will reap the benefits from these 10 steps for many decades to come.

1. Commit to planning

Planning is the key to dietary success – have the foods you need on hand to eat well most of the time. Planning ensures that you will typically have healthy meals and won't get stuck without the right protein-rich snack choices to support your level of activity or training. Take control of your food and your nutrition simply by setting aside 20 to 30 minutes each week to plan your meals and snacks for the week ahead. This may include some meal prep, shopping or making a meal plan – whatever helps make smart nutrition choices easy amid a busy life.

2. Commit to breakfast balance

A strong nutrition foundation comes from prioritising a protein- and fibre-rich breakfast to give your metabolic rate a boost, provide essential nutrients and keep you full and satisfied, ideally until lunchtime. A protein-rich breakfast is crucial as it helps regulate the hormones that keep us feeling full and satis-fied, meaning we're less likely to overeat later in the day. Turn to trusty favourites such as eggs, baked beans, cottage cheese, protein powder and natural yoghurt. After a decent sleep, the earlier you have your breakfast, the better it is for metabolism. Make it a priority to avoid refined carbohydrates and sugary breakfast on-the-go options such as large slices of Turkish toast, muffins, banana bread, juices and large, sweet milky coffees.

3. Commit to eating more vegetables

One of the most powerful things you can do to improve your nutrient intake and digestive health and support weight control is to eat lower calorie, nutrient-dense salad and vegetables each day. This means making sure that you add fresh food to each meal and snack, and aiming for at least a couple of cups of salad and/or vegetables at main meals.

4. Commit to the best quality carbs

Carbohydrates play an important role in optimally fuelling the muscles and the brain but the type of carbs we choose is important. Wholegrain and wholefood varieties of carbohydrates – whether rice, noodles, pasta, bread or starchy vegetables – are always a much better choice nutritionally than refined and processed varieties like white bread, white rice, processed types of potato such as chips, and fruit that has been made into snacks. Variety with your carbs is also important to support digestive health, so make it a focus to seek out different options at mealtimes and not repeat the same carbs day in and day out. If you like stir-fry for dinner, try serving it with brown rice, quinoa, black rice, a brown-rice noodle or some lentil pasta.

5. Commit to good quality protein

Protein-rich foods such as lean meat, seafood, eggs, dairy, legumes and soy-based foods not only add key nutrients such as calcium, iron, zinc and omega-3 fat to the diet, but they also play a key role in regulating appetite, and as such, getting adequate amounts of protein at each meal and snack helps to keep calorie intake controlled throughout the course of the day. Aiming for one protein-rich food at each meal and snack will help you to reach your daily protein targets.

6. Commit to avoiding sugary drinks

Juices, soft drinks, cordials, vitamin waters and energy drinks are generally just sugar-based fluids, which few of us need. Not only are liquid calories less likely to be accounted for, leaving us vulnerable to consuming too many calories when we drink them, but they are also highly acidic and not great for our teeth. Focus your fluid intake on water only and be mindful that milk-based coffees such as lattes also contain calories and hence cannot be consumed freely.

7. Commit to not wasting your calories

There is nothing wrong with enjoying more indulgent foods occasionally, but the daily consumption of high-calorie processed fast food, snacks, chocolates, biscuits and pastries will not only increase your intake of ultra-processed foods, but also make it difficult to lose body fat. If you are routinely eating these calorie-dense foods, which are easy to overeat, losing weight becomes much harder. Focus on enjoying your favourite foods occasionally, or a more indulgent meal once or twice a week, and prioritising your nutritional foundation the rest of the time to support sustainable fat loss long term.

8. Commit to less alcohol

There is nothing wrong with enjoying a drink or two on occasion but a habit of drinking 3 to 4 glasses of wine a night, or binge drinking on weekends, can be hard to break and has many negative impacts. Not only does alcohol have almost as many calories as fat, but when you are drinking your body is so busy processing the alcohol that you are likely to be storing any food calories that you consume while you are drinking.

9. Commit to compensation

You are human – there will always be times when you overdo it, whether it is at a special occasion or simply because you are craving higher fat, higher calorie foods. The secret to balancing some food indulgences with weight control long term is learning to compensate when you have overdone things – to eat a lighter meal if you have overeaten, or eat more soups and salads and skip the alcohol for a period of time if you have had several days of overdoing it. Regular monitoring of your weight will also ensure that you are aware when things may be starting to creep up so you can pull back when necessary.

10. Commit to quality over quantity

Perhaps one of the strongest nutritional messages that will benefit you throughout life is to always aim for quality over quantity when it comes to your food choices. Go for an amazing homemade hamburger rather than a fast-food meal, the best quality Belgian chocolate rather than the 2-for-1 bars at the service station, and a little French cheese or pâté rather than half a block of cheddar. Each time you go to over-indulge, ask yourself, 'Is this really worth it?' If the answer is no, you will find it easier to cut back when you need to and indulge a little when it really is worth it.

Successful and sustainable fat loss does not have to be about extreme diets and restriction. Rather, the science of fat loss is about creating a consistent calorie deficit via a meal plan that you genuinely like and enjoy so that it is sustainable. In Burn we have shown you the easy ways to build your own sustainable fat-loss plan using our simple fat-loss formula so you can kiss diets and deprivation goodbye for good.

Move the right way

While this is primarily a book on diet (we are dietitians after all), it is impossible to write a book on sustainable fat loss without factoring in a discussion on movement and exercise (yes, they are different things). Indeed, when it comes to fat metabolism, calorie intake is important but so too is increasing metabolism and teaching the body to burn calories more efficiently over time, which is largely dependent on how much and the type of exercise we are doing. So, let's start with the importance of moving and why it's necessary to accept that moving is just what we need to do to keep our body healthy.

It's time to stop thinking and start moving

How much time over the course of your adult life have you spent thinking about what you 'should' be doing when it comes to exercise? After countless hours (and much money) on trainers, gym memberships, exercise equipment, classes you are probably still not moving enough. It is time to accept that moving our body every day and exercising regularly to keep fit is something we all need to do to be our best and healthiest selves. It is time to get on with it.

Just move

The human body is programmed to move, a lot. As soon as we get the movement we require each day, not only does it help us to burn more calories, but our mood, digestion, hormones, energy levels and cravings are all positively impacted. The issue, of course, is that modern life is not overly conducive to moving a lot, with most of us spending much of the day sitting.

For this reason, if you are not a natural mover, the best thing you can do to support your fat-loss goals is to move as much as you can each day. A small walk each morning will not be enough; rather, we need regular increments of incidental movement as well as our daily steps to prevent weight gain, let alone support fat loss – remember, bodies are supposed to move.

Then, add in the exercise

If you manage to move your body each day, and also have time to exercise, getting your heart rate up 3 to 4 times each week with a fast walk or run, trip to the gym for resistance training, bike ride or personal training session will benefit your metabolism, or the body's ability to efficiently burn calories long term. The key with training is to get your heart rate up, and to mix it up regularly to continue to challenge the body, build muscle and efficiently burn calories.

Also, keep in mind that while forms of exercise like Pilates and swimming are great for toning, flexibility and mental health, they are not as good at burning calories and supporting an increase in metabolic function as high-intensity cardio and resistance training is.

How to find time to exercise

For busy women, adding more and more into already overfull schedules is not ideal and not usually sustainable as life routinely gets in the way. A more sustainable, less pressurised approach can be to gradually factor in more movement over time, so it does not add more stress to an already stressful life.

1) Start with steps

Getting to the gym for a workout or going for an extra run is indeed a luxury and generally depends on several factors coming together each day (partner arriving home on time, children are happy and well, et cetera) but if you can simply start to monitor your steps on a daily basis, research shows that we will automatically increase our movement by as much as 2000 steps each day, simply by being more mindful of our movement choices each day.

2) Planning is key

Life is very busy, so unless we actively plan, even occasionally, to exercise, get to the gym, meet a friend for a walk instead of a coffee or a drink, it will never happen. Start by planning a session, even a walk for just 20 to 30 minutes once or twice a week, and you will be surprised how quickly you will find yourself looking for those opportunities to get to the gym or move your body, simply because you feel so much better after doing it.

3) Build your network

It is much easier to keep a commitment to exercise when you have others to do it with. In busy lives, we are often surprisingly isolated from others as we spend more time online and less in face-to-face interaction, reducing our quality time with others as we are so distracted by technology. Coming together with friends or even family to move or exercise is not only a motivator itself, but means you are also getting support and quality time with those around you while getting your exercise in.

4) Make it easy

How many people do you know who have a gym membership but rarely go? Or have exercise equipment they never use? Or, have intentions to get up each morning and walk, but never do? If you are not a natural mover, you have to make it as easy as possible to do it. If that means hiring a bike or a treadmill so you can exercise at home in front of the TV, or paying someone to train you at the gym so you turn up, or accepting you will never go to the gym and therefore cancelling your membership and accepting that walking needs to be your exercise of choice, just do it.

5) Enrol in events

Some people are more social than others, and as such, the thought of spending an hour alone at the gym is less than appealing; on the other hand, training with others or having an event to prepare for is all they need to keep them interested and moving regularly. Whether you need to join a bike or walking club, or initiate group registrations for big walking, running or cycling events, group training or participation may be just what you need to get some exercise consistency in your life.

Are you training or maintaining?

Just as mixing up our food benefits our metabolism, so too does mixing up our exercise. Many of us find ourselves doing the exact same type of exercise at exactly the same time each day, and wonder why our body is no longer changing. If you are walking the same route at the same time each day, or doing the same exercise class each week that you have been doing for the past 5 years, chances are that your body has grown so used to your exercise routine that you barely break a sweat, and this is likely to be one of the reasons you are not getting the weight-loss results you are expecting.

To burn a significant number of calories and increase metabolic rate over time you need to make sure that at least some of your exercise is challenging the body. This means your heart rate needs to be elevated and you need to be slightly breathless for at least some of the workout. In many cases you will find that once you shift your exercise from maintaining to training, you will again start to see changes in your body size and fitness.

Meet Penny: the benefits of changing up your exercise routine and eating for fat loss

Penny was 39 and, by most definitions, quite healthy. Over the years, however, her weight had slowly crept up by 5 kilograms, despite her not changing her nutrition and even taking up daily Pilates sessions where she had once been quite sedentary. Though she was someone who ate well and stayed active she wasn't seeing the changes she hoped for.

Penny had suffered from gestational diabetes and had a family history of diabetes. She was in close contact with her doctor, who had told her that her blood-glucose levels were slowly creeping up over time, despite her body weight remaining healthy.

Penny came to see her dietitian for 3 reasons: to reduce her diabetes risk long term, to lose the 5 kilograms that had snuck on over the years and to gain some lean muscle mass (in her words, 'tone up more'). She was sick and tired of 'doing everything right' only to find she never actually got any traction towards her goals.

Working with her dietitian, Penny learnt that overall, her meals were healthy but they often lacked enough fibre and veggie bulk for fullness. Her carbs were too high for her requirements and her protein was too low at breakfast, but too high at dinner. These changes were easy enough to fix with some personalised advice and only required slight adjustments to her usual meals.

Her dietitian also referred her to an exercise physiologist, who wrote her a new strength-training program she could do in her home gym. Penny swapped her daily Pilates for 3 weight-based strength sessions a week, one or two HIIT-based sessions to get her heart rate higher, and still kept up with her Pilates on the other day or two. She also implemented a 10-minute post-dinner walk with her family to help with blood sugar regulation.

Penny also learnt her carbs were too high for the type of exercise she was doing, but adding in more strength training and HIIT-based training instead of Pilates meant her muscles were more receptive to the carbs. A slight carb reduction with her meals supported her further towards her goals. Whereas previously she had avoided snacking due to her goal of fat loss, building in a balanced afternoon snack assisted Penny to reduce the mindless snacking on the kids' dinner while she waited for her husband to come home from work. The afternoon snack also helped to better fuel her more intense workouts.

The results were nothing short of remarkable. Overall, Penny lost 6.5 kilograms in 4 months, dropped 6 centimetres from her waist measurement and increased her strength and cardiovascular fitness overall. Her whole family benefited from the extra veggies with meals and the bonding time that their after-dinner walk provided. Her doctor told her that her diabetes risk had been reduced and her 3-monthly blood-glucose average had started to trend down. Penny's results are a testament to the power of small but personalised changes, and show that while healthy eating and eating for fat loss may seem similar, they require different strategies and attention to detail. Her example also shows the power of working within a multi-disciplinary team (dietitian, doctor and exercise physiologist).

Let's talk about . . . energy balance

We've all heard time and time again that energy balance is all about 'energy in and energy out' or 'calories in and calories out'. In other words: if the energy that you 'put in' (the food you eat) matches the energy you 'put out' (the exercise/activity that you do), then your body stays at the same weight (weight maintenance). If your 'energy in' is larger than your 'energy out' then you'll gain weight. If your 'energy out' is larger than your 'energy in' then you'll lose weight. Sounds simple enough, but in fact, these elements have a lot of intricacies.

COMMON FACTORS THAT INFLUENCE THE 'ENERGY IN' AND 'ENERGY OUT' EQUATION

FACTORS THAT INFLUENCE THE ENERGY THAT GOES INTO OUR BODY	FACTORS THAT INFLUENCE THE ENERGY THAT COMES OUT OF OUR BODY
Hormones, appetite and satiety	Genetics and body size
Macronutrient intake	Energy burned at rest and dieting history
Energy density of foods consumed and eating meals out	Exercise
Portion sizes and grazing/snacking	Age and metabolism
Absorption	Incidental movement
Psychological factors (sleep, stress, mindset, self-sabotage, emotional eating)	Energy burned through processing food

A few factors that people tend to overlook (and that can be hugely helpful!) when it comes to losing weight are:

Incidental activity

Classified as the movement your body does each day that isn't formal exercise – for example, taking the stairs, getting up off the couch to find the remote, pacing your office on a work call, et cetera. If you have a desk job and sit down for the majority of the day, this becomes even more important. Often, a daily 30- to 45-minute workout for weight loss isn't enough if you then sit for 8 to 9 hours the rest of the day. Some extra steps most days will generally make weight loss far easier if you have a sedentary job or lifestyle.

Food absorption

We recommend a higher protein diet for weight loss as of the 3 macronutrients (protein, fats and carbohydrates), the body uses the most energy to break down protein. As discussed in food sequencing, it may also help increase satiety to support weight-loss goals. We also recommend a focus on wholefoods as they take more energy to break down than ultra-processed foods.

Age

From the age of 30, muscle mass decreases by approximately 3 to 8 per cent per decade, and after the age of 60 this rate of decline increases.[109] Muscle is a metabolic tissue so the more you have, the faster your metabolism and the easier it is to lose weight.

Hormonal status

As you enter peri-menopause your hormones start to fluctuate, which can impact weight gain and cause a loss of muscle tissue. Therefore, weight training a minimum of twice a week becomes even more important past 40 years of age.

Sleep

Lack of sleep can cause a spike in cortisol, which can lead to shifts in body composition. A lack of sleep can also cause the hormone leptin to become reduced (leptin tells the body when you've had enough to eat and helps to regulate long-term energy balance).[110] So, we recommend you stop scrolling on your phone at night and start prioritising a good night's sleep.

Metabolic adaptation

After a period of dieting, the body tends to down-regulate its processes and your basal metabolic rate drops, which makes it difficult to continue to lose weight and follow the same plan that originally worked for you.

NOTES FROM THE NUTRITION COUCH
WEIGHT-LOSS PLATEAUS – HOW DO YOU DEAL WITH THEM?

It can be easy to feel discouraged on your weight-loss journey if there isn't a shift on the scales each day. It can feel tempting to give up at this point but try reframing it as the final challenge.

To be clear, a weight-loss plateau isn't something that happens in the short term – it happens after several weeks, if not months. That's partly why, as a general rule, weighing yourself daily is not helpful. Twice a week at most is ideal to see a trend on the scale and give you some indication of how you are progressing.

We see a lot of clients who may be close to their goal but need that extra help to get over the final hurdle. The good news is that with some small changes and some specific attention to certain areas, you may be able to get past that pesky plateau.

Go back to basics and consider the variables that are going on – as we discussed in previous chapters, hunger and the makeup of our meals can play a significant role.

1. **Ensure you are being consistent.** The large majority of weight-loss plateaus we see in our clinics are due to a lack of consistency with eating and exercise. Clients get complacent and

214

little things creep in one by one. They don't seem like a lot but just 10 to 20 per cent more in your meals can be the difference between losing and maintaining weight.

2. **Check your hunger.** Less hunger is not necessarily a good sign on your weight-loss journey. If you're not hungry 3 to 4 hours after a balanced meal, that could suggest your metabolism has started to down-regulate. A change in nutrients, meal composition or meal timing may be the ideal next step.

3. **Variety of diet.** Are you eating the same thing every day? Our bodies can get used to the same foods quickly, so it may be as simple as adjusting the ingredients or the carbohydrate and protein levels of your breakfast.

4. **Check your exercise.** Look closely at your heart rates if you use a fitness tracker and consider whether your exercise method of choice is elevating your heart rate. If it's not, try upping the intensity in a few workouts each week.

26 April 2023[111]

Why am I not losing weight?

There are many reasons weight loss may slow or plateau when you are following a program designed to support fat loss. Firstly, keep in mind that a week of no loss is nothing to be concerned about – that is a normal part of the weight-loss process and should be expected. However, if you have been following a plan and there has been no change for several weeks, there are several variables that could be impacting your results.

Start with the food
Are you eating too much?
It may be that your portions are too large, or that you are mindlessly munching on extras. If you feel that you are truly compliant

with your program, it may be time to take a closer look at what is really going on. While we don't advocate constant monitoring, in short bursts of focus, it can be really helpful to gauge where you're at. Spend a day or two writing down everything you eat and drink, and popping it into a calorie-monitoring program like MyFitnessPal if you have time. Keeping track will show you exactly how many calories you are consuming in reality and allow you to adjust accordingly.

Are you eating enough carbs?

While getting enough calories is one thing, the macro balance you consume is also important. Too few carbs for your age, metabolism and level of activity mean the body will not have enough fuel to actively metabolise fat and, over time, weight loss may slow. A small female needs at least 80 to 100 grams of carbs, if not more, that being at least 30 per cent of overall calorie intake. If your carb intake is routinely low, or less than 100 grams, it may be worth increasing it a little to see if that stimulates appetite and metabolism and supports fat loss.

Are you not eating enough?

While tight restriction can induce relatively quick weight loss, over time it is entirely possible to be eating too little to support fat metabolism. One of the reasons for this is that as you lose weight – specifically body fat – your cells often become more sensitive to the hormones that control fat metabolism, which means you burn calories more efficiently. Over time, this means you may need to eat more (not less). So if your regular daily calorie intake is 1200 and your weight loss has slowed, try increasing your daily food intake slowly over time.

Is your timing off?

Meal timing is important and if you routinely eat your first meal after 9 am, push lunch back to mid-to-late afternoon and/or eat dinner earlier, yours may be less than ideal. If you have less than 10 to 12 hours without food overnight, you may not be maximising your metabolic rate and this may be slowing fat loss. Aim to have your first meal before 8 am, lunch by 12 noon and your final food of the day by no later than 7 or 8 pm. The more calories you consume in the first half of the day, and the lighter your diet at night, the better for fat loss.

Are you over-indulging on weekends?

Weekends are tricky when you are actively trying to lose weight. The lack of daily structure coupled with celebrations, socialising, catch-ups and parties can mean that a whole lot of extra calories can slip in, without us noticing any real change with our intake or appetite. Plus, it can be tricky to get your regular amount of exercise when the days are filled with kids' sport and other social commitments. If you know you tend to overdo things on the weekend, it may be time to cut back on the social events and pay a lot more attention to what you are eating for a weekend or two, to see if cutting back a little on the weekend is the missing link for your weight loss.

Next, look at exercise
Are you moving enough?

Modern life means we move a whole lot less than we ever used to and unfortunately for many of us it simply won't be enough to go for a walk each day and get the basic amount of movement we need for health, let alone weight loss. Even if you are getting a decent number of steps each day, if you then spend the remainder of your day sitting, this may explain why the scales have become stagnant. Try mixing things up by changing the times you walk and the intensity you walk at. It is much better to break the movement up throughout the day than to walk once then remain sedentary for hours at a time.

Are you training with intention?

It is not uncommon to see clients who are exercising regularly but have got to a point in their program where they are no longer challenging their muscles to an extent that they are efficiently burning extra calories. The human body is exceptionally smart, and what may yield good fat-loss results initially will need to be regularly adjusted to continue to increase metabolic rate and to burn as many calories as that same exercise once did. The key here is to routinely change gym programs, walking and running routes, and types of training to continue getting the 'training and burning' effect of exercise, rather than maintaining.

Or is it something else?

Your mindset

Your attitude towards lifestyle changes can play a surprisingly large role in your success. If you feel annoyed, frustrated, resentful or even angry about your positive lifestyle changes, it can subconsciously be undermining your efforts. For example, if you feel annoyed that you have to work so much harder than everyone else when it comes to weight control, so you don't follow the plan 100 per cent, or if the general annoyance you carry means that every action step you take is laborious, this will undermine your general commitment and attitude. If you do not like the plan or program you are following, the key is to develop one that you genuinely like and that fits in with you, or you will never fully commit and always find yourself falling short of the outcomes you desire.

Hormones

There are several signs and symptoms that your weight loss may be impacted by variables such as hormones, which may be largely out of your control. Extreme fatigue, cravings, unexpected weight gain, bad skin, irregular periods, unusual changes in mood and energy levels may be all signs that it is time to make a trip to your doctor and take a closer look at your blood markers of key hormones that can impact weight loss including thyroid hormones, insulin and oestrogen.

Medication

There are a range of different medications including contraceptives and anti-depressants that can directly and indirectly impact weight control by influencing both appetite and metabolism. If you suspect that a medication is directly impacting your ability to be diet compliant, or resulting in weight gain in a way that feels beyond your control, schedule time to discuss it with your doctor and see if there may be better alternatives when it comes to weight control.

COMMON MISTAKES THAT INHIBIT FAT LOSS

Achieving a calorie deficit to consistently lose weight or lose body fat is not without its challenges. Not only does strong nutritional knowledge come into play but so do our behaviours, habits, consistency, exercise, hormones and social supports.

However, when you know what the common hurdles are, it's much easier to look out for and avoid them. Below is a list of the most common mistakes we tend to see when it comes to losing weight or reducing body fat. We don't usually observe people doing all of these things at once, more likely just a few, but they are enough to be the difference between losing weight and maintaining it.

- Eating too many healthy fats.
- Eating the same thing all the time.
- Portion sizes are too big.
- Exercising the same way all the time.
- Eating off the kids' plates.
- Eating 'back' the calories burned through exercise.

- Skipping meals then over-grazing.
- Not eating enough vegetables.
- Not moving enough/desk job.
- Eating out too much.
- Too many unsustainable 'quick fixes/fad diets'.
- Lack of consistency.
- Blowing out on the weekends.
- Drinking too much alcohol.
- Eating too many commercially processed 'health-food' products.
- Not getting enough sleep.
- Not eating enough protein and fibre at meals.
- Eating healthily but not in a calorie deficit.
- Intermittent fasting but eating too much in the fasting window.
- Drinking too many calories, e.g. sweetened coffees, juices, smoothies, bubble tea.

The end, but not goodbye

As we finish up this book, we want to remind you that this may be the end of the book, but it is certainly not goodbye. Our chart-topping podcast, *The Nutrition Couch*, has over 5 million downloads and is the top nutrition podcast in Australia. It's available on all large podcast-streaming platforms and has hundreds of episodes in the back catalogue. If you would like to follow our Instagram or Facebook social media pages, please head to @the_nutrition_couch_podcast to give us a follow, and to look at our website, please head to www.thenutritioncouch.com.

Final word

If you are looking to lose weight and keep it off long term, acceptance and action are key. You can read every nutrition, exercise and motivation book that exists, but you will never change if you don't take action towards your goals. So, do it now! Grab a pen and paper and write down a list of things that you simply need to accept as part of your new healthy lifestyle. Next, write down a list of things that you need to take action on right now, this month, this year and in the future. Start working towards that list today because your future self will be so grateful that you started today, and you never quit.

Remember, in a couple of years, it won't matter how long it took you. You'll just be grateful that you read this book, that you took massive action, that you believed in yourself and that you started and never stopped. We know it feels hard and overwhelming but just start, somewhere, anywhere and JUST DON'T QUIT!

RECIPES
&
MEAL
PLANS

Apple Crumble Bowls
Makes 2

NOURISH

Prep time: 10 minutes
Cooking time: 20 minutes

Ingredients:

2 small green apples, peeled, cored, chopped

2 teaspoons lemon juice

1 teaspoon unsalted butter

½ teaspoon ground cinnamon

2 tablespoons natural almonds, chopped

¼ teaspoon ground cinnamon

1 tablespoon softened unsalted butter

Crumble:

½ cup (50 g) rolled oats

1 tablespoon wholemeal flour

2 tablespoons brown sugar

To serve:

320 g low-fat high-protein yoghurt (plain or vanilla flavoured)

Method:

1. Preheat oven to 180°C. Place apples in a medium bowl. Drizzle over the lemon juice and set aside.
2. Melt the butter in a medium saucepan over medium heat. Add the apples and cinnamon and cook, stirring occasionally, for 5 minutes or until apples are just softened. Set aside.
3. To make the crumble, combine the oats, flour, sugar, almonds and cinnamon in a medium bowl. Add the butter and rub into flour mixture using fingertips until mixture resembles coarse crumbs.
4. Lightly spray two ½ cup (125 ml) capacity ovenproof ramekins with olive oil. Divide apple mixture between ramekins and top with crumble mixture. Bake for 20 minutes or until topping is golden.
5. Serve crumbles with the yoghurt.

Per serve:

21.1 g protein

19.8 g fat (7.7 g saturated fat)

50.9 g carb

7.2 g dietary fibre

2007 kJ (480 cals)

Vegetable Hash Browns with Eggs
Serves 2

Prep time: 12 minutes
Cooking time: 10 minutes

Ingredients:

½ cup (75 g) coarsely grated sweet potato

1 small zucchini, coarsely grated

¼ golden shallot, finely chopped

1 tablespoon coarsely chopped dill

5 eggs

2 teaspoons cornflour

1½ tablespoons extra-virgin olive oil

2 small (about 40 g each) slices multigrain sourdough bread, toasted

1 cup (45 g) baby spinach leaves

8 cherry tomatoes

50 g marinated (or soft) goat's cheese

pinch of dried chilli flakes, to serve (optional)

Method:

1. Combine the sweet potato, zucchini, shallot and dill in a medium bowl. Season with salt and freshly ground black pepper. Add one egg and the cornflour to the vegetable mixture and stir to combine.

2. Heat 1 tablespoon of the oil in a large non-stick frying pan over medium heat. Form vegetable mixture into 6 patties and add to hot pan. Cook for 2–3 minutes each side or until golden and cooked through. Transfer to a plate.

3. Heat remaining oil in same pan over medium heat. Fry remaining eggs until cooked to your liking. Divide vegetable hash, toast, eggs, spinach and tomato between two serving plates. Serve with goat's cheese and sprinkle with chilli flakes (if using). Season to taste with salt and freshly ground black pepper.

Per serve:

25.7 g protein

32.4 g fat (8.8 g saturated fat)

29.4 g carb

5.5 g dietary fibre

2177 kJ (521 cals)

Higher Protein Avo Smash
Serves 1

Prep time: 10 minutes
Cooking time: not required

Ingredients:

¾ cup (110 g) frozen podded
    edamame, thawed
½ clove garlic, crushed
½ firm ripe avocado, stone removed,
    peeled

2 teaspoons lime juice
1 large (about 60 g) slice multigrain
    sourdough bread
25 g feta cheese, crumbled
1 tablespoon dill sprigs

Method:

1. Place edamame in a medium bowl and mash with a fork. Add garlic, avocado and lime juice and continue to mash until well combined, keeping some texture.
2. Toast bread and top with avocado mixture, feta and dill sprigs.

Per serve:

26.1 g protein
20.5 g fat (6.0 g saturated fat)
45.4 g carb

14.6 g dietary fibre
2055 kJ (492 cals)

Protein Berry Pancakes

Serves 1

NOURISH

Prep time: 5 minutes
Cooking time: 10–15 minutes

Ingredients:

1 egg

¼ cup (60 ml) skim milk

⅓ cup (55 g) wholemeal flour

½ teaspoon baking powder

½ teaspoon ground cinnamon

1 tablespoon vanilla whey protein
    powder

1 tablespoon extra-virgin olive oil

½ cup (75 g) mixed frozen berries

1 tablespoon reduced-fat ricotta
    cheese, to serve

1 teaspoon sugar-free maple syrup,
    to serve (optional)

Method:

1. Place egg and milk in a medium bowl and whisk until combined. Whisk in flour, baking powder, cinnamon and protein powder until well combined and smooth.

2. Heat the oil in a large non-stick frying pan over medium heat. Ladle ¼ cup (60 ml) amounts of batter into pan. Cook pancakes for 2–3 minutes each side, or until golden and cooked through.

3. Meanwhile, place frozen berries in a microwave-safe dish, cover and microwave on high for 30 seconds or until warmed through.

4. Serve pancakes topped with ricotta, warm berries and maple syrup (if using).

Per serve:

25.3 g protein

24.8 g fat (4.6 g saturated fat)

41.7 g carb

9.3 g dietary fibre

2139 kJ (512 cals)

Mediterranean Tuna Pasta Bake

Serves 4

Prep time: 15 minutes
Cooking time: 25 minutes

Ingredients:

180 g dried pulse pasta

1 teaspoon extra-virgin olive oil

250 g mushrooms, sliced

400 g tin diced tomatoes

½ cup (125 ml) tomato passata

425 g tin tuna in spring water, drained, flaked

2 large zucchini, cut into 3 cm pieces

1 large red capsicum, deseeded, chopped

80 g pitted kalamata olives, halved

20 g (¼ cup) fresh wholemeal breadcrumbs (see tip)

120 g reduced-fat feta cheese, crumbled, to serve

fresh basil leaves, to serve (optional)

Method:

1. Preheat oven to 180°C. Lightly spray an 8 cup (2 litre) capacity ovenproof baking dish with olive oil.
2. Cook pasta in a large saucepan of lightly salted boiling water according to packet instructions or until al dente. Drain.
3. Meanwhile, heat oil in a medium frying pan over high heat. Cook mushrooms, stirring occasionally, for 2–3 minutes or until golden.
4. Combine pasta, diced tomatoes and passata in prepared baking dish. Add mushrooms, tuna, zucchini, capsicum and olives and stir to combine. Season with salt and freshly ground black pepper. Sprinkle with breadcrumbs.
5. Bake for 20 minutes or until pasta bake is golden and bubbling. Serve topped with feta and basil (if using).

Tip: Fresh breadcrumbs are best made from stale bread (about 3 days old). Process bread, with or without crusts, until coarse crumbs form. Alternatively, you can use store-bought (dried) breadcrumbs.

Per serve:

42.5 g protein

14.6 g fat (4.7 g saturated fat)

39.9 g carb

9.9 g dietary fibre

2061 kJ (493 cals)

Veggie-packed Sausage Rolls

Serves 4 (Makes 16 sausage rolls)

Prep time: 25 minutes
Cooking time: 35 minutes

Ingredients:

1 tablespoon extra-virgin olive oil

1 small brown onion, finely chopped

4 cloves garlic, crushed

1 small carrot, peeled, coarsely grated

1 small zucchini, coarsely grated

100 g cup mushrooms, coarsely chopped

400 g tin brown lentils, rinsed, drained

2 tablespoons dried Italian herbs

120 g grated 25% reduced-fat cheddar cheese

2 sheets frozen light puff pastry, just thawed

1 egg, lightly beaten

1 tablespoon sesame seeds, to sprinkle

healthy tomato relish, to serve (optional)

Method:

1. Preheat oven to 180°C. Line two baking trays with baking paper.
2. Heat the oil in a large non-stick frying pan over medium heat. Add the onion and cook, stirring, for 3–4 minutes or until softened. Add garlic and cook, stirring, for 30 seconds or until fragrant. Add the carrot, zucchini and mushrooms and cook, stirring often, for 5 minutes or until vegetables are soft and any liquid has evaporated.
3. Stir in the lentils and herbs. Season to taste with salt and freshly ground black pepper. Transfer to a large heatproof bowl. Set aside to cool slightly, then stir through the grated cheese.
4. Cut each pastry sheet in half. Place one quarter of the veggie mixture in a log shape along one long edge of the pastry. Brush the opposite edge with egg. Roll up tightly to enclose. Repeat with the remaining pastry and filling. Cut each roll into 4 pieces, score with a knife and place, seam side down, on the prepared trays.

5. Brush the pastry tops with remaining egg and sprinkle with sesame seeds. Bake for 25 minutes or until rolls are puffed and golden. Allow to cool slightly before serving with a big side salad to add nutrients and volume to the meal and tomato relish (if using).

Per serve:

22.3 g protein

24.6 g fat (12.7 g saturated fat)

51.4 g carb

6.7 g dietary fibre

2219 kJ (531 cals)

Quick and Healthy Fried Rice
Serves 4

Prep time: 10 minutes
Cooking time: 15 minutes

Ingredients:

2 eggs

500 g extra-lean minced pork

1 brown onion, finely chopped

2 cups (260 g) frozen peas, corn and carrot mix

2 zucchini, finely diced

1 large red capsicum, deseeded, finely chopped

2 cups (330 g) cooked brown basmati rice, slightly cooled

2 tablespoons salt-reduced soy sauce

3 tablespoons oyster sauce

1 tablespoon sesame oil

sliced spring onion and long red chilli, to serve (optional)

Method:

1. Whisk the eggs together in a medium bowl and set aside.
2. Lightly spray a wok or large frying pan with olive oil and heat over high heat. Add pork and stir-fry, using a wooden spatula to break up mince, for 3–4 minutes or until browned.
3. Add onion and stir-fry for 2 minutes. Add frozen vegetables, zucchini and capsicum and stir-fry for 4–5 minutes or until vegetables are almost tender. Push the vegetable mixture to one side of the pan and pour in eggs. Scramble eggs using a spatula and then stir through the vegetable mixture. Add rice, sauces and sesame oil and stir-fry until hot and vegetables are just tender.
4. Serve sprinkled with spring onion and chilli (if using).

Per serve:

36.0 g protein

14.8 g fat (3.6 g saturated fat)

44.2 g carb

7.2 g dietary fibre

1967 kJ (471 cals)

Zesty Chicken Tacos
Serves 4

Prep time: 15 minutes
Cooking time: 12 minutes

Ingredients:

400 g chicken breast tenderloins

30 g salt-reduced taco seasoning

1 tablespoon extra-virgin olive oil

400 g tin black beans, rinsed, drained

1 mango, stone removed, peeled, diced

¼ red onion, finely diced

2 tablespoons chopped coriander, plus extra whole leaves, to serve

juice of 1 lime

3 cups (240 g) shredded red cabbage

12 corn taco shells

Method:

1. Place chicken on a clean board or plate. Sprinkle taco seasoning evenly over chicken to coat. Heat oil in a large non-stick frying pan on medium–high heat. Cook chicken for 3–4 minutes each side or until chicken is golden and cooked through. Transfer chicken to a clean board and cut into 3–4 cm pieces.

2. To make the salsa, combine black beans, mango, onion, chopped coriander and lime juice in a medium bowl. Season with salt and freshly ground black pepper and stir to combine.

3. Divide cabbage, chicken and salsa between taco shells. Serve topped with extra coriander leaves.

Per serve:

31.8 g protein

14.3 g fat (2.5 g saturated fat)

44.3 g carb

10.6 g dietary fibre

1880 kJ (450 cals)

Chicken Parmi, Chips and Salad

Serves 4

Prep time: 20 minutes
Cooking time: 40 minutes

Ingredients:

500 g washed potatoes (or sweet potato), cut into 1–2 cm thick chips

2 tablespoons extra-virgin olive oil

½ cup (35 g) fresh multigrain breadcrumbs (see tip)

¼ cup (20 g) finely grated parmesan cheese

1 teaspoon dried Italian herbs

2 eggs

2 large (about 200 g each) chicken breasts, halved horizontally

1 cup (250 ml) tomato passata

80 g grated mozzarella cheese

Method:

1. Preheat oven to 200°C. Line two baking trays with baking paper.
2. To make the chips, place potatoes, 1 tablespoon oil and a pinch of salt in a large bowl and toss to coat potatoes evenly in the oil. Arrange chips in a single layer on one of the prepared trays and bake for 30 minutes, turning chips halfway through cooking time, or until golden and crisp.
3. Meanwhile, combine breadcrumbs, parmesan and herbs in a shallow bowl and season with salt and freshly ground black pepper. Whisk eggs together in a separate shallow bowl.
4. Using a meat mallet, pound chicken breasts to flatten slightly. Working one at a time, dip the chicken in the egg mixture, allowing excess to drain, then cover in crumb mixture, making sure both sides are evenly coated.
5. Heat remaining oil in a large non-stick frying pan over medium–high heat. Cook chicken, in batches if necessary, for 2–3 minutes each side or until golden. Transfer the chicken to second baking tray and bake for 10 minutes or until cooked through. In the final 2 minutes of cooking, remove chicken and top with passata and mozzarella. Return to oven and continue to bake until mozzarella is melted and golden.
6. Top parmi with basil and serve with baked chips and a big side salad of your choosing.

Tip: Fresh breadcrumbs are best made from stale bread (about 3 days old). Process bread, with or without crusts, until fine crumbs form. Alternatively you can use store-bought (dried) breadcrumbs.

Per serve:

36.7 g protein

19.7 g fat (6.4 g saturated fat)

23.2 g carb

4.3 g dietary fibre

1786 kJ (427 cals)

Nourishing Beef and Veggie Lasagne

Serves 6

Prep time: 20 minutes
Cooking time: 1 hour, 30 minutes

Ingredients:

400 g peeled pumpkin, thinly sliced

3 zucchini, thinly sliced lengthways

1 teaspoon extra-virgin olive oil

1 onion, finely chopped

4 cloves garlic, crushed

1 teaspoon ground cumin

500 g extra-lean minced beef

2 carrots, peeled, grated

2 sticks celery, finely chopped

400 g tin brown lentils, rinsed,
    drained

400 g tin diced tomatoes

40 g butter

⅓ cup (50 g) plain flour

2 cups (500 ml) skim milk

6 fresh (47 g each) lasagne sheets

¾ cup (65 g) grated 25% reduced-
    fat cheddar cheese

fresh basil leaves, to serve (optional)

Method:

1. Preheat oven to 180°C. Line two baking trays with baking paper and lightly spray a 16 cup (4 litre) capacity ovenproof dish with olive oil. Arrange pumpkin and zucchini in a single layer on prepared trays. Lightly spray with olive oil and bake for 20 minutes or until tender. Set aside.

2. Meanwhile, heat oil in a large non-stick frying pan over medium heat. Add onion and cook, stirring occasionally, for 5 minutes or until softened. Add garlic and cumin and cook, stirring, for 30 seconds or until fragrant. Increase heat to high and add mince. Cook, breaking mince up with a wooden spoon, for 7–8 minutes or until browned. Add carrot, celery, lentils and tomato and stir to combine. Reduce heat to low and simmer, uncovered, for a further 5–7 minutes, or until slightly reduced. Season with salt and freshly ground black pepper to taste. Remove from heat and set aside.

3. Melt butter in a medium saucepan over low heat. Add flour and stir to combine. Slowly add milk, stirring constantly until smooth and well combined. Continue to cook, stirring, for 8–10 minutes or until mixture is

thick enough to coat the back of a spoon. Season to taste with salt and freshly ground black pepper.

4. Place a third of the meat sauce in the base of the prepared dish. Top with a third of the vegetables and 2 pasta sheets. Top with a third of the white sauce. Repeat layers twice more, finishing with a layer of white sauce. Sprinkle top with grated cheese.

5. Bake for 35–45 minutes or until top is golden and lasagne is cooked through. Serve with a big side salad to increase the volume and nutrients in the meal.

Per serve:

36.9 g protein

17.1 g fat (7.6 g saturated fat)

52.8 g carb

9.9 g dietary fibre

2234 kJ (534 cals)

Vegetable Egg Bites

Serves 4 (3 egg bites per serve)

Prep time: 10 minutes
Cooking time: 25 minutes

Ingredients:

8 eggs

1 cup (250 g) reduced-fat cottage cheese

2 spring onions, white parts only, thinly sliced

12 cherry tomatoes, quartered

1 cup (45 g) baby spinach leaves

1 cup (185 g) fresh or frozen corn kernels

2 tablespoons chopped flat-leaf parsley

½ cup (55 g) grated mozzarella cheese

Method:

1. Preheat oven to 180°C and lightly spray 12 holes of a ½ cup (125 ml) capacity muffin tin with olive oil.
2. Whisk the eggs together in a large bowl. Stir in the cottage cheese and season to taste with salt and freshly ground black pepper.
3. Lightly spray a medium non-stick frying pan with olive oil and heat over high heat. Add the spring onions and cook, stirring, for 1 minute. Add tomatoes and spinach and cook, stirring occasionally, for a further 2 minutes or until the spinach is wilted. Stir through the corn and parsley.
4. Divide the vegetable mixture among the muffin holes. Pour over the egg mixture.
5. Top each egg bite with a sprinkle of cheese and bake for 15–20 minutes or until they are golden, puffed and just firm to touch. Serve with side salad.

Per serve:

27.6 g protein

15.8 g fat (6.6 g saturated fat)

10.1 g carb

2.1 g dietary fibre

1260 kJ (301 cals)

Banana and Almond Protein Smoothie
Makes 1

Prep time: 5 minutes

Ingredients:

1 banana, cut into chunks, frozen

1 tablespoon almond butter

20 g vanilla whey protein powder

1 cup (250 ml) unsweetened
calcium-fortified almond milk

10 ice cubes

Method:

Place all ingredients in a blender and blend until smooth. Drink immediately.

Per serve:

25.5 g protein

13.2 g fat (1.1 g saturated fat)

22.0 g carb

6.0 g dietary fibre

1357 kJ (325 cals)

Overnight Berry Bircher
Serves 1

Prep time: 10 minutes

Ingredients:

⅓ cup (35 g) rolled oats

½ small zucchini, finely grated

2 teaspoons chia seeds

¼ cup (60 ml) milk of choice

½ cup (120 g) low-fat high-protein vanilla yoghurt

1 teaspoon sugar-free maple syrup (optional)

½ cup (75 g) blueberries

sprinkle of pepita seeds, to serve (optional)

Method:

Combine oats, zucchini, chia seeds, milk, yoghurt and maple syrup (if using) in a container with a lid. Stir until well combined, cover and refrigerate overnight. In the morning, top with blueberries and pepitas (if using).

Per serve:

19.9 g protein

5.8 g fat (1.0 g saturated fat)

35.8 g carb

9.0 g dietary fibre

1226 kJ (293 cals)

Mexican Eggs with Beans
Serves 4

Prep time: 10 minutes
Cooking time: 35 minutes

Ingredients:

1 tablespoon extra-virgin olive oil

1 brown onion, finely chopped

½ teaspoon dried chilli flakes, plus extra to serve

1 teaspoon smoked paprika

1 red capsicum, deseeded, chopped

400 g tin red kidney beans, rinsed, drained

400 g tin diced tomatoes

8 eggs, at room temperature

1 avocado, stone removed, peeled, sliced

½ cup coriander leaves

Method:

1. Preheat oven to 180°C.
2. Heat oil in a large (30 cm diameter) non-stick ovenproof frying pan over medium heat. Add onion and cook, stirring, for 5 minutes or until softened. Add chilli flakes and paprika and cook, stirring, for 30 seconds or until fragrant. Add capsicum, kidney beans and tomatoes. Cook, stirring occasionally, for 2–3 minutes, then reduce heat to low and simmer, uncovered, for 10 minutes or until mixture has thickened.
3. Make 4 indents in the bean mixture and break two eggs into each indent. Transfer pan to oven and bake for 15 minutes or until eggs are cooked to desired consistency.
4. Serve topped with avocado, coriander and an extra sprinkle of chilli flakes.

Per serve:

20.6 g protein

19.3 g fat (4.0 g saturated fat)

17.9 g carb

10.7 g dietary fibre

1461 kJ (349 cals)

Breakfast Nourish Bowl
Serves 1

Prep time: 10 minutes

Ingredients:

200 g low-fat high-protein Greek yoghurt

1 cup (about 150 g) chopped seasonal fruit

1 tablespoon LSA (ground linseeds, sunflower seeds & almonds)

1 tablespoon pepitas

Method:

Place yoghurt in a bowl. Top with fruit and sprinkle with LSA and pepitas.

Per serve:

25.3 g protein

11.4 g fat (1.5 g saturated fat)

21.5 g carb

7.4 g dietary fibre

1280 kJ (306 cals)

Chicken Tenders with Slaw

Serves 4

BURN

Prep time: 25 minutes
Cooking time: 15 minutes

Ingredients:

2 eggs
¼ cup (60 ml) water
¾ cup (55 g) breadcrumbs (see tip)
400 g chicken tenderloins
lemon wedges, to serve (optional)

Slaw:
2 teaspoons lemon juice
¼ cup (60 ml) extra-virgin olive oil

2 tablespoons Greek yoghurt
¼ red cabbage, coarsely chopped
¼ white cabbage, coarsely
   chopped
1 carrot, peeled, coarsely grated
2 spring onions, white parts only,
   thinly sliced

Method:

1. Preheat oven to 200°C. Place an oven-safe baking rack on a rimmed baking tray. Lightly spray rack with olive oil spray.
2. Whisk eggs and water together in a shallow bowl. Place breadcrumbs in a second shallow bowl. Season with salt and freshly ground black pepper.
3. Working one at a time, dip the tenderloins into the egg mixture, then press into the breadcrumb mixture to coat evenly. Place tenderloins on prepared rack, spray lightly with olive oil and bake for 10–15 minutes, turning halfway through cooking time, or until golden and cooked through.
4. Meanwhile, to make the slaw, combine juice, olive oil and yoghurt in a large bowl. Add cabbages, carrot and spring onions and toss to lightly coat in the dressing.
5. Divide tenderloins and slaw between serving plates and serve with lemon wedges (if using) and some extra yoghurt.

Tip: To make fresh breadcrumbs, process stale bread in a food processor to form fine crumbs. Alternatively, use store-bought (dried) breadcrumbs.

Per serve:

29.9 g protein
21.7 g fat (4.1 g saturated fat)
11.4 g carb

5.4 g dietary fibre
1552 kJ (371 cals)

Smoked Salmon and Ricotta Edamame Pasta

Serves 2

Prep time: 10 minutes
Cooking time: 25 minutes

Ingredients:

200 g dried edamame pasta

2 teaspoons extra-virgin olive oil

1 bunch broccolini, halved

½ cup (80 g) frozen peas

100 g smoked salmon, torn into bite-sized pieces

100 g reduced-fat ricotta cheese

250 g cherry tomatoes, halved

2 teaspoons finely grated parmesan cheese

lemon wedges, to serve

Method:

1. Cook pasta in a large saucepan of lightly salted boiling water following packet instructions or until al dente. Drain.

2. Meanwhile, heat oil in a medium non-stick frying pan over high heat. Add broccolini and cook, stirring occasionally, for 3–4 minutes or until tender-crisp. Transfer broccolini to a plate and keep warm.

3. Add peas to same pan and cook over medium heat, stirring occasionally, for 3–4 minutes or until almost tender. Reduce heat to low and add drained pasta, smoked salmon and ricotta. Stir to combine and cook for 2–3 minutes or until hot. Add tomatoes and cook for a further 2–3 minutes.

4. Season with freshly ground black pepper. Serve pasta sprinkled with parmesan and with the broccolini and lemon wedges on the side.

Per serve:

38.7 g protein

19.8 g fat (6.4 g saturated fat)

12.6 g carb

13.3 g dietary fibre

1711 kJ (409 cals)

Pulled Pork Mexican Bowl
Serves 4

Prep time: Overnight for the pork + 20 minutes
Cooking time: 7–8 hours

Ingredients:

2 tablespoons Mexican seasoning

400 g boneless pork shoulder, excess fat trimmed

2 vine-ripened tomatoes, chopped

½ red onion, finely diced

4 cups (240 g) shredded iceberg lettuce

1 cup (185 g) tinned corn kernels rinsed, drained

1 cup (170 g) tinned black beans, rinsed, drained

½ cup (40 g) 25% reduced-fat cheddar cheese, grated

1 avocado, stone removed, peeled, diced

¼ cup (70 g) Greek yoghurt

¼ cup store-bought tomato salsa

2 tablespoons chopped coriander

lime wedges, to serve

Method:

1. Rub the Mexican seasoning into the pork shoulder. Cover pork loosely with plastic film and refrigerate for a minimum of 2 hours or overnight.
2. The next morning, preheat oven to 230°C and bring the pork to room temperature. Place pork in a shallow roasting dish and roast, uncovered, for 30 minutes or until pork starts to brown. Reduce oven to 120°C and continue to roast, uncovered, for 7–8 hours or until middle of pork registers 82°C on a meat thermometer and meat feels tender throughout. Remove from the oven and set aside to cool before shredding pork with two forks. Discard any fatty bits.
3. To serve, combine tomato and red onion in a medium bowl. Divide lettuce, pork, tomato mixture, corn, black beans, cheese and avocado between serving bowls. Top with a dollop of yoghurt and salsa. Serve with a sprinkle of coriander and lime wedges.

Per serve:

28.1 g protein

14.1 g fat (4.5 g saturated fat)

26.4 g carb

9.3 g dietary fibre

1505 kJ (360 cals)

Teriyaki Salmon with Asian Greens
Serves 2

Prep time: 40 minutes
Cooking time: 20 minutes

Ingredients:

2 x 120 g salmon fillets

1 bunch baby bok choy, trimmed

1 bunch gai laan (Chinese broccoli), trimmed

1 tablespoon oyster sauce

2 teaspoons sesame seeds

2 spring onions, green part only, thinly sliced, to serve

sliced long red chilli, to serve

Marinade:

1 teaspoon teriyaki sauce

1 tablespoon salt-reduced soy sauce

1 tablespoon rice wine vinegar

1 teaspoon honey

1 teaspoon sesame oil

3 cloves garlic, crushed

1 teaspoon finely grated ginger

Method:

1. Combine all marinade ingredients in a shallow dish. Add salmon and turn to coat. Cover and marinate in fridge for at least 30 minutes.
2. Preheat oven to 200°C and line a baking tray with baking paper. Place salmon on prepared tray and bake for 12–15 minutes or until cooked to your liking.
3. Meanwhile, heat a wok or large non-stick frying pan over high heat. Stir-fry bok choy, gai laan and oyster sauce for 3–4 minutes or until vegetables are tender-crisp. Add a dash of water to wok if needed.
4. Divide salmon and greens between serving plates. Sprinkle with sesame seeds, spring onion and chilli to serve.

Per serve:

33.7 g protein

18.9 g fat (3.6 g saturated fat)

11.2 g carb

6.9 g dietary fibre

1514 kJ (360 cals)

Salt and Pepper Tofu with Wombok Salad
Serves 4

BURN

Prep time: 30 minutes
Cooking time: 10 minutes

Ingredients:

600 g firm tofu

¼ cup (50 g) cornflour

¾ teaspoon ground black pepper

¾ teaspoon ground white pepper

¾ teaspoon sea salt

½ teaspoon Chinese five spice

2 tablespoons extra-virgin olive oil

sliced long red chilli and spring
   onions, to serve (optional)

Salad:

8 cups (640 g) shredded wombok

1 bunch small radishes, thinly
   sliced

1 continental cucumber, halved,
   thinly sliced

1 carrot, peeled, cut into thin
   matchsticks

1 cup mint leaves, chopped

1 cup coriander leaves,
   chopped

Dressing:

3 cloves garlic, crushed

2 tablespoons lime juice

1 tablespoon rice wine vinegar

2 tablespoons fish sauce

2 teaspoons white sugar

½ cup (125 ml) cold water

Method:

1. Wrap the tofu in paper towel. Place a clean board on top of tofu, and then top with a couple of tins (to weigh tofu down). Set aside for 10 minutes to remove excess water, changing paper towel if it becomes very wet.

2. Cut the tofu into cubes. Combine cornflour, pepper, salt and five spice on a large plate. Toss each piece of tofu in spice mixture to coat evenly.

3. Heat oil in a large non-stick frying pan over medium–high heat. Cook tofu, in batches, for 3–5 minutes, turning occasionally, or until golden and crisp. Transfer to a plate.

4. To make the salad, place wombok, radish, cucumber, carrot and herbs in a large bowl.

5. To make the dressing, place all ingredients in a jar with a lid and shake well to combine. Add dressing to salad and toss to combine.
6. Serve tofu with salad, sprinkled with chilli and spring onions (if using).

Per serve:

23.2 g protein

20.7 g fat (3.0 g saturated fat)

14.8 g carb

12.0 g dietary fibre

1517 kJ (363 cals)

Garlic Prawn Cauli Risotto

Serves 2

BURN

Prep time: 10 minutes
Cooking time: 25 minutes

Ingredients:

1 tablespoon extra-virgin olive oil

250 g cup mushrooms, chopped

1 cup (150 g) frozen green peas

1 zucchini, sliced

4 cups (420 g) fresh or frozen cauliflower rice

1 tablespoon cornflour

½ cup (125 ml) salt-reduced chicken stock

¼ cup (20 g) finely grated parmesan cheese

4 cloves garlic, crushed

12 large green prawns, peeled, deveined, tails on

finely chopped fresh parsley, to serve

Method:

1. Heat 2 teaspoons oil in a large heavy-based saucepan or pan over medium heat. Cook mushrooms, peas and zucchini, stirring, for 3–4 minutes or until vegetables are tender and mushrooms start to brown. Season with salt and freshly ground black pepper.

2. Reduce the heat to medium–low, add the cauliflower and toss to coat. Add the stock a few tablespoons at a time, stirring until stock is absorbed after each addition.

3. When the cauliflower is beginning to soften, add remaining stock, cover and continue to cook for 2 minutes, or until cauliflower is tender.

4. Place cornflour and 1 tablespoon water in a small bowl and stir until smooth. Add cornflour mixture and simmer until reduced and slightly thickened. Add a little more stock if needed.

5. Stir in the parmesan cheese and season to taste with salt and freshly ground black pepper. Remove from heat and set aside.

6. Meanwhile, heat remaining oil in a medium non-stick frying pan over medium heat. Cook garlic, stirring, for 30 seconds or until fragrant. Add prawns and cook, stirring occasionally, until golden and cooked through.

7. To serve, spoon risotto into bowls, top with prawns and sprinkle with parsley.

Per serve:

39.7 g protein

14.6 g fat (3.6 g saturated fat)

19.2 g carb

11.0 g dietary fibre

1656 kJ (396 cals)

Crumbed Fish Bites and Veggie Chips

Serves 4

BURN

Prep time: 20 minutes

Cooking time: 40 minutes

Ingredients:

500 g firm white fish fillets

¼ cup (40 g) plain flour

1 cup (70 g) fresh multigrain breadcrumbs (see tip)

1 egg

⅓ cup (25 g) finely grated parmesan cheese

1 tablespoon extra-virgin olive oil

1 teaspoon garlic powder

1 teaspoon dried oregano

2 large carrots, peeled, cut into 2 cm thick chips

2 large zucchini, cut into 2 cm thick chips

lemon wedges and tzatziki, to serve

Method:

1. Preheat oven to 200°C. Place an oven-safe baking rack on a rimmed baking tray and spray with olive oil. Line a second baking tray with baking paper.
2. Pat fish dry with paper towel. Season with salt and freshly ground black pepper and cut into 3 cm cubes.
3. Place flour on a large plate and breadcrumbs on a second large plate. Place egg in a shallow bowl and whisk with a fork until lightly beaten. Toss each cube of fish into the flour, shaking off any excess, then coat in the egg and finally in the breadcrumbs until evenly coated.
4. Place fish on prepared rack and bake for 15–20 minutes, turning halfway through cooking time, or until golden and cooked through
5. Meanwhile, combine parmesan, oil, garlic powder and oregano in a large bowl. Add carrot and zucchini chips and toss to coat in the parmesan mixture. Arrange chips on second prepared tray in a single layer. Bake for 15–20 minutes, turning chips halfway through cooking time, or until golden and crisp.
6. Serve fish bites and veggie chips with a dollop of tzatziki, a wedge of lemon and a side salad.

Tip: Fresh breadcrumbs are best made from stale bread (about 3 days old). Process bread, with or without crusts, until fine crumbs form. Alternatively you can use store-bought (dried) breadcrumbs.

Per serve:

34.3 g protein

15.4 g fat (3.7 g saturated fat)

24.7 g carb

6.4 g dietary fibre

1628kJ (389 cals)

Zucchini and Ricotta Fritters
Serves 4

Prep time: 20 minutes
Cooking time: 10–15 minutes

Ingredients:

3 large zucchini

1½ cups (375 g) reduced-fat ricotta cheese

¾ cup (120 g) wholemeal plain flour

2 large eggs

½ cup (40 g) grated 25% reduced-fat cheddar cheese

2 spring onions, white parts only, thinly sliced

2 cloves garlic, crushed

finely grated zest of ½ lemon

1 teaspoon baking powder

1 tablespoon extra-virgin olive oil

sliced spring onions, green parts only, to serve

Method:

1. Coarsely grate the zucchini and place in a sieve. Using paper towel, press on zucchini to remove excess liquid.
2. Place drained zucchini, 1 cup (250 g) ricotta, flour, eggs, cheese, spring onion, garlic, zest and baking powder in a large bowl. Mix until well combined. Using clean hands, shape mixture into 12 fritters.
3. Heat the oil in a large non-stick frying over medium–high heat. Cook fritters, in batches, for 2–3 minutes each side or until golden and cooked through. Transfer to a plate lined with paper towel to drain any excess oil.
4. Serve fritters with a dollop of remaining ricotta and sprinkle with extra spring onions. Add a big side salad to your serving.

Per serve:

20.0 g protein

14.4 g fat (5.5 g saturated fat)

24.6 g carb

6.5 g dietary fibre

1371 kJ (328 cals)

Beef San Choy Bow
Serves 4

Prep time: 20 minutes
Cooking time: 10 minutes

Ingredients:

1 tablespoon sesame oil

500 g extra-lean minced beef

225 g tin water chestnuts, drained, chopped

2 spring onions, white parts only, finely chopped

1 cup (110 g) coarsely grated carrot

1 cup (130 g) coarsely grated zucchini

1 red capsicum, deseeded, diced

1 cup finely chopped cup mushrooms

400 g tin baby corn spears, drained, chopped

2 tablespoons hoisin sauce

1 tablespoon salt-reduced soy sauce

12 cos lettuce leaves

1 tablespoon sesame seeds

1 cup (55 g) trimmed bean sprouts

thinly sliced spring onion, green parts only, to serve

thinly sliced long red chilli, to serve (optional)

Method:

1. Heat oil in a wok or large non-stick frying pan over high heat. Add the mince and stir-fry, breaking mince up with a wooden spatula, for 3–4 minutes or until mince starts to brown. Add chestnuts, white spring onion, carrot, zucchini, capsicum, mushrooms and corn and stir-fry for 2 minutes. Add hoisin and soy sauce and stir-fry for a further 1–2 minutes or until hot and vegetables are just tender-crisp.

2. Spoon mixture into cos lettuce leaves and top with sesame seeds, bean sprouts, green spring onion and chilli (if using).

Per serve:

34.3 g protein

13.5 g fat (3.9 g saturated fat)

18.1 g carb

7.8 g dietary fibre

1430 kJ (342 cals)

Capsicum Beef Stir-fry with Cauli Rice
Serves 4

BURN

Prep time: 15 minutes
Cooking time: 10 minutes

Ingredients:

1 tablespoon extra-virgin olive oil

500 g lean beef stir-fry strips,
    fat trimmed

1 brown onion, thinly sliced

2 cloves garlic, crushed

1 large carrot, peeled, thinly sliced

1 red capsicum, deseeded, sliced

250 g cup mushrooms, sliced

2 tablespoons oyster sauce

1 tablespoon salt-reduced soy sauce

4 cups (420 g) cauliflower rice,
    cooked, to serve

½ cup (80 g) roasted cashews,
    to serve

Method:

1. Heat the oil in wok or large frying pan over high heat. Stir-fry the beef in two batches for 2 minutes or until browned. Remove from the wok and set aside.

2. Return wok to a high heat. Add onion and garlic and stir-fry for 1–2 minutes. Add carrot, capsicum and mushrooms and stir-fry for 2–3 minutes or until vegetables are just tender-crisp.

3. Return the beef to the wok with the oyster sauce and soy sauce and stir-fry until hot and well combined. Serve with cauliflower rice, topped with cashews and spring onions.

Per serve:

40.9 g protein

15.5 g fat (3.0 g saturated fat)

18.9 g carb

8.3 g dietary fibre

1663 kJ (398 cals)

Nourish 7-day Meal Plan

	BREAKFAST	MORNING TEA
DAY 1	2-egg vegetable omelette with wholegrain toast	150 g high-protein yoghurt + 1 piece of fruit
DAY 2	Apple Crumble Bowls (page 225)	1 small milky coffee + 2 small protein balls
DAY 3	Eggs on toast with tomatoes and spinach	150 g high-protein yoghurt + 1 piece of fruit
DAY 4	Higher Protein Avo Smash (page 227)	20 g cheese + 4 wholegrain crackers + 1 tomato, sliced
DAY 5	Overnight oats with high-protein yoghurt and banana	1 small milky coffee + 25 g roasted chickpeas
DAY 6	Vegetable Hash Browns with Eggs (page 226)	20 g cheese + 4 wholegrain crackers + 1 tomato, sliced
DAY 7	Protein Berry Pancakes (page 228)	1 apple + 1 tbsp peanut butter

LUNCH	AFTERNOON TEA	DINNER
Veggie-packed Sausage Rolls (page 230)	25 g roasted chickpeas + 2 squares dark chocolate	Mediterranean Tuna Pasta Bake (page 229)
Mediterranean Tuna Pasta Bake (page 229)	30 g mixed nuts + 2 cups of air-popped popcorn	Quick and Healthy Fried Rice (page 232)
Quick and Healthy Fried Rice (page 232)	2 corn thins + 4 tbsp cottage cheese + 1 tomato, sliced + basil	Chicken Parmi, Chips and Salad (page 234)
Jacket potato topped with tinned tuna + bowl of salad or soup	150 g high-protein yoghurt + 1 piece of fruit	150 g grilled salmon + 2 cups roasted vegetables
Soup and sandwich: 1 cup pumpkin soup + 50 g ham, 1 slice cheese, ½ tomato, 2 slices wholegrain bread	30 g mixed nuts + 20 g cheese + small piece of fruit	Zesty Chicken Tacos (page 233)
6-8 pieces sashimi, 1 cup edamame, small seaweed salad	2 small protein balls	Nourishing Beef and Veggie Lasagne (page 236)
Chicken and salad wrap + bowl of vegetable soup or side salad with avocado	30 g mixed nuts + 2 cups of air-popped popcorn	Veggie-packed Sausage Rolls (page 230)

Burn 7-day Meal Plan

	BREAKFAST	MORNING TEA
DAY 1	Banana and Almond Protein Smoothie (page 239)	Small milk coffee + small apple
DAY 2	Breakfast Nourish Bowl (page 242)	150 g high-protein yoghurt + small banana
DAY 3	Vegetable Egg Bites (page 238)	2 small protein balls
DAY 4	Overnight Berry Bircher (page 240)	Small milk coffee + small pear
DAY 5	Vegetable Egg Bites (page 238)	1 boiled egg + veggie sticks + 1 tablespoon hummus
DAY 6	Banana and Almond Protein Smoothie (page 239)	150 g high-protein yoghurt + small banana
DAY 7	Mexican Eggs with Beans (page 241)	Small milk coffee + small protein ball

LUNCH	AFTERNOON TEA	DINNER
Zucchini and Ricotta Fritters (page 253) with salad	30g mixed nuts + 20 g cheese	Teriyaki Salmon with Asian Greens (page 246)
Tuna and salad wrap + bowl of vegetable soup	1 slice cheese + 2 grain crackers + veggie sticks	Pulled Pork Mexican Bowl (page 245)
Smoked Salmon and Ricotta Edamame Pasta (page 244)	100 g high-protein yoghurt + 10 nuts + 1 piece of fruit	Capsicum Beef Stir-fry with Cauli Rice (page 255)
Pulled Pork Mexican Bowl (page 245)	2 small protein balls	Salt and Pepper Tofu with Wombok Salad (page 247)
Beef San Choy Bow (page 254)	1 slice cheese + 2 grain crackers + veggie sticks	Crumbed Fish Bites and Veggie Chips (page 251)
Toasted cheese and tomato sandwich on protein bread + bowl of vegetable soup	2 small protein balls	Garlic Prawn Cauli Risotto (page 249)
Chicken Tenders with Slaw (page 243)	100 g high-protein yoghurt + 10 nuts + 1 fruit	Zucchini and Ricotta Fritters (page 253) with salad

NOTES

Unless otherwise stated, all links were accessed June 2024.

1   The Nutrition Couch (2023). The Psychological Impact of "Diet Culture". Diet and Lifestyle Post Menopause. Are Low Sugar Foods Better For Us? 18 July 2023. omny.fm/shows/the-nutrition-couch/the-psychological-impact-of-diet-culture-diet-and

2   Evert, A. B., & Franz, M. J. (2017). Why Weight Loss Maintenance Is Difficult. *Diabetes spectrum: a publication of the American Diabetes Association*, *30*(3), 153–156. doi:10.2337/ds017-0025

3   Harvard Health Publishing. (n.d.) 'Diet & Weight Loss', Harvard Medical School, health.harvard.edu/topics/diet-and-weight-loss

4   LaGreca, M., Hutchinson, D., & Barry, L. (2020). A Multi-Faceted Approach to Weight Loss: A Case Report. *Integrative medicine 19*(1), 38–45.

5   Harvard Medical School. (n.d.) What are ultra-processed foods and are they bad for our health? *Harvard Health Blog*. health.harvard.edu/blog/what-are-ultra-processed-foods-and-are-they-bad-for-our-health-2020010918605

6   Gardner, B., Lally, P., & Wardle, J. (2012). Making health habitual: the psychology of 'habit-formation' and general practice. *The British Journal of General Practice: the journal of the Royal College of General Practitioners*, *62*(605), 664–666. doi:10.3399/bjgp12X659466

7   Butryn, M. L., Phelan, S., Hill, J. O., & Wing, R. R. (2007). Consistent self-monitoring of weight: a key component of successful weight loss maintenance. *Obesity (Silver Spring, Md.), 15*(12), 3091–3096. doi: 10.1038/oby.2007.368

8   Benn, Y., Webb, T. L., Chang, B. P., & Harkin, B. (2016). What is the psychological impact of self-weighing? A meta-analysis. *Health psychology review, 10*(2), 187–203. doi:10.1080/17437199.2016.1138871

9   Berry, R., Kassavou, A., & Sutton, S. (2021). Does self-monitoring diet and physical activity behaviors using digital technology support adults with obesity or overweight to lose weight? A systematic literature review with meta-analysis. *Obesity reviews : an official journal of the International Association for the Study of Obesity, 22*(10), e13306. doi:10.1111/obr.13306

10   The Nutrition Couch (2022). Orthorexia, What Is It and What are Orthorexia's Indicators? "Sequential Eating", Does It Have Any Benefits? Which Supplements Can Best Combat a Cold or Flu?, 3 July 2022. omny.fm/shows/the-nutrition-couch/orthorexia-what-is-it-and-what-are-orthorexias-ind

11   McCarthy, Mary & Collins, Alan & Flaherty, Sarah Jane & McCarthy, Sinéad. (2017). Healthy eating habit: A role for goals, identity, and self-control? *Psychology & Marketing, 34*, 772–785. doi:10.1002/mar.21021

12   De Ridder, D., & Gillebaart, M. (2017). Lessons learned from trait self-control in well-being: making the case for routines and initiation as important components of trait self-control. *Health Psychology Review, 11*(1), 89–99. doi:10.1080/17437199.2016.1266275

13   Frank, P., Jokela, M., Batty, G. D., Lassale, C., Steptoe, A., & Kivimäki, M. (2022). Overweight, obesity, and individual symptoms of depression: A multicohort study with replication in UK Biobank. *Brain, behavior, and immunity, 105*, 192–200. doi:10.1016/j.bbi.2022.07.009

14   U Paixão, C., Dias, C. M., Jorge, R., Carraça, E. V., Yannakoulia, M., de Zwaan, M., Soini, S., Hill, J. O., Teixeira, P. J., & Santos, I. (2020). Successful weight loss maintenance: A systematic review of weight control registries. *Obesity reviews: an official journal of the International Association for the Study of Obesity, 21*(5), e13003. doi: 10.1111/obr.13003

15 Luszczynska, A., Sobczyk, A., & Abraham, C. (2007). Planning to lose weight: randomized controlled trial of an implementation intention prompt to enhance weight reduction among overweight and obese women. *Health psychology: official journal of the Division of Health Psychology, American Psychological Association, 26*(4), 507–512. doi:10.1037/0278-6133.26.4.507

16 Hill, E. B., Cubellis, L. T., Wexler, R. K., Taylor, C. A., & Spees, C. K. (2023). Differences in Adherence to American Heart Association's Life's Essential 8, Diet Quality, and Weight Loss Strategies Between Those With and Without Recent Clinically Significant Weight Loss in a Nationally Representative Sample of US Adults. *Journal of the American Heart Association, 12*(8), e026777. doi:10.1161/ JAHA.122.026777

17 Australian Government Dept Health and Aged Care (n.d.) Physical activity and exercise guidelines for all Australians for Adults (18 to 64 years), health.gov.au/topics/physical-activity-and-exercise/ physical-activity-and-exercise-guidelines-for-all-australians/ for-adults-18-to-64-years

18 Koliaki, C., Spinos, T., Spinou, M., Brinia, M. E., Mitsopoulou, D., & Katsilambros, N. (2018). Defining the Optimal Dietary Approach for Safe, Effective and Sustainable Weight Loss in Overweight and Obese Adults. *Healthcare (Basel, Switzerland), 6*(3), 73. doi:10.3390/ healthcare6030073

19 Christakis, N. A., & Fowler, J. H. (2007). The spread of obesity in a large social network over 32 years. *The New England journal of medicine, 357*(4), 370–379. doi:10.1056/NEJMsa066082

20 The Nutrition Couch (2023). Telltale Signs of Fixed Mindsets. Reviewing a New No Added Sugar Chocolate Milk. Susie's Winter Warming Spinach Pie Recipe. 24 May 2023. omny.fm/shows/the- nutrition-couch/telltale-signs-of-fixed-mindsets-reviewing-a- new-n

21 Appleton J. (2018). The Gut-Brain Axis: Influence of Microbiota on Mood and Mental Health. *Integrative medicine (Encinitas, Calif.), 17*(4), 28–32.

22 Liangpunsakul, S. (2010). Relationship between alcohol intake and dietary pattern: findings from NHANES III. *World journal of gastroenterology, 16*(32), 4055–4060. doi:10.3748/wjg.v16.i32.4055

McLean, C., Ivers, R., Antony, A., McMahon, A. (2024) Malnutrition, nutritional deficiency and alcohol: A guide for general practice. *Australian Journal of General Practitioners*, 53(4), April 2024. doi:10.31128/AJGP-05-23-6827

23   Bishehsari, F., Magno, E., Swanson, G., Desai, V., Voigt, R. M., Forsyth, C. B., & Keshavarzian, A. (2017). Alcohol and Gut-Derived Inflammation. *Alcohol research: current reviews*, 38(2), 163–171, PMID: 28988571

24   Viola Helaakoski, Jaakko Kaprio, Christer Hublin, Hanna M Ollila, Antti Latvala, Alcohol use and poor sleep quality: a longitudinal twin study across 36 years, *SLEEP Advances*, Volume 3, Issue 1, 2022, zpac023, doi:10.1093/sleepadvances/zpac023

25   Australian Government Dept Health and Aged Care (n.d.) How much alcohol is safe to drink? health.gov.au/topics/alcohol/about-alcohol/how-much-alcohol-is-safe-to-drink

26   Mouri, M.I., Badireddy, M. (2023)Hyperglycemia. StatPearls Publishing, ncbi.nlm.nih.gov/books/NBK430900/

27   Ludwig, D. S., & Ebbeling, C. B. (2018). The Carbohydrate-Insulin Model of Obesity: Beyond "Calories In, Calories Out". *JAMA internal medicine*, *178*(8), 1098–1103. doi:10.1001/jamainternmed.2018.2933

28   The Nutrition Couch (2023). The Psychological Impact of "Diet Culture". Diet and Lifestyle Post Menopause. Are Low Sugar Foods Better For Us? 18 June 2023. omny.fm/shows/the-nutrition-couch/the-psychological-impact-of-diet-culture-diet-and

29   Mouri, M.I., Badireddy, M. (2023)Hyperglycemia. StatPearls Publishing, ncbi.nlm.nih.gov/books/NBK430900/

30   Tardy, A. L., Pouteau, E., Marquez, D., Yilmaz, C., & Scholey, A. (2020). Vitamins and Minerals for Energy, Fatigue and Cognition: A Narrative Review of the Biochemical and Clinical Evidence. *Nutrients*, *12*(1), 228. doi:10.3390/nu12010228

31   Coad, J., & Conlon, C. (2011). Iron deficiency in women: assessment, causes and consequences. *Current opinion in clinical nutrition and metabolic care*, *14*(6), 625–634. doi:10.1097/MCO.0b013e32834be6fd

32   Tardy, A. L., Pouteau, E., Marquez, D., Yilmaz, C., & Scholey, A. (2020). Vitamins and Minerals for Energy, Fatigue and Cognition: A Narrative Review of the Biochemical and Clinical Evidence. *Nutrients*, *12*(1), 228. doi:10.3390/nu12010228

33   Dr. Anis Rehman, A. & PachecoStaff, (2024). Do Women Need More Sleep Than Men? *Sleep Foundation*, 15 March 2024, sleepfoundation. org/women-sleep/do-women-need-more-sleep-than-men

34   The Nutrition Couch (2023) The Best and Worst High Protein Breads. How to Pick a Good Meal Kit. Is Chia a Good Breakfast Option? 1 October 2023. omny.fm/shows/the-nutrition-couch/ the-best-and-worst-high-protein-breads-how-to-pick

35   Campbell, W. W., Deutz, N. E. P., Volpi, E., & Apovian, C. M. (2023). Nutritional Interventions: Dietary Protein Needs and Influences on Skeletal Muscle of Older Adults. *The journals of gerontology. Series A, Biological sciences and medical sciences*, *78*(Suppl 1), 67–72. doi:10.1093/gerona/glad038

36   Schoenfeld, B. J., & Aragon, A. A. (2018). How much protein can the body use in a single meal for muscle-building? Implications for daily protein distribution. *Journal of the International Society of Sports Nutrition*, *15*(10). doi:10.1186/s12970-018-0215-1

37   Eat for Health (n.d.) Nutrient Reference Values for Australia and New Zealand. eatforhealth.gov.au/nutrient-reference-values/nutrients/ protein

38   Lonnie, M., Hooker, E., Brunstrom, J. M., Corfe, B. M., Green, M. A., Watson, A. W., Williams, E. A., Stevenson, E. J., Penson, S., & Johnstone, A. M. (2018). Protein for Life: Review of Optimal Protein Intake, Sustainable Dietary Sources and the Effect on Appetite in Ageing Adults. *Nutrients*, *10*(3), 360. doi:10.3390/nu10030360

39   Weijzen, M. E. G., Kouw, I. W. K., Geerlings, P., Verdijk, L. B., van Loon, L. J. C. (2020). During hospitalization, older patients at risk for malnutrition consume <0.65 grams of protein per kilogram body weight per day. *Nutrition in Clinical Practice*, *35*(4), 655–663. doi: 10.1002/ncp.10542

40   Malesza, I. J., Malesza, M., Walkowiak, J., Mussin, N., Walkowiak, D., Aringazina, R., Bartkowiak-Wieczorek, J., & Mądry, E. (2021). High-Fat, Western-Style Diet, Systemic Inflammation, and Gut Microbiota: A Narrative Review. *Cells*, *10*(11), 3164. doi:10.3390/cells10113164

41   DiNicolantonio, J. J., & O'Keefe, J. H. (2017). Good Fats versus Bad Fats: A Comparison of Fatty Acids in the Promotion of Insulin Resistance, Inflammation, and Obesity. *Missouri medicine*, *114*(4), 303–307.

42 Simopoulos A. P. (2002). The importance of the ratio of omega-6/omega-3 essential fatty acids. *Biomedicine & pharmacotherapy, 56*(8), 365–379. doi:10.1016/s0753-3322(02)00253-6

43 Calder P. C. (2010). Omega-3 fatty acids and inflammatory processes. *Nutrients, 2*(3), 355–374. doi:10.3390/nu2030355

44 Dugan, C., Simpson, A., Peeling, P., Lim, J., Davies, A., Buissink, P., MacLean, B., Jayasuriya, P., & Richards, T. (2023). The Perceived Impact of Iron Deficiency and Iron Therapy Preference in Exercising Females of Reproductive Age: A Cross-Sectional Survey Study. *Patient preference and adherence, 17*, 2097–2108. doi:10.2147/PPA.S397122

45 Beckett, J. M., & Ball, M. J. (2015). Zinc status of northern Tasmanian adults. *Journal of nutritional science, 4*, e15. doi:10.1017/jns.2015.12

46 Henry, M. J., Pasco, J. A., Nicholson, G. C., Seeman, E., & Kotowicz, M. A. (2000). Prevalence of osteoporosis in Australian women: Geelong Osteoporosis Study. *Journal of clinical densitometry: the official journal of the International Society for Clinical Densitometry, 3*(3), 261–268. doi:10.1385/jcd:3:3:261

47 Rohm, T.V., Meier, D.T., Olefsky, J.M., Donath, M.Y. (2022) Inflammation in obesity, diabetes, and related disorders, *Immunity, 55*(1), 31-55. doi:10.1016/j.immuni.2021.12.013

48 Thyroid Foundation (n.d.) Thyroid Facts: Iodine Deficiency and Nutrition, thyroidfoundation.org.au/Iodine-Deficiency
Australian Bureau of Statistics (2013) Iodine, 11 December 2013, abs.gov.au/articles/iodine

49 Australian Thyroid Foundation (n.d.) Iodine deficiency & nutrition. thyroidfoundation.org.au/Iodine-Deficiency

50 Ioniță-Mîndrican, C. B., Ziani, K., Mititelu, M., Oprea, E., Neacșu, S. M., Moroșan, E., Dumitrescu, D. E., Roșca, A. C., Drăgănescu, D., & Negrei, C. (2022). Therapeutic Benefits and Dietary Restrictions of Fiber Intake: A State of the Art Review. *Nutrients, 14*(13), 2641. doi:10.3390/nu14132641

51 Fayet-Moore, F., Cassettari, T., Tuck, K., McConnell, A., & Petocz, P. (2018). Dietary Fibre Intake in Australia. Paper II: Comparative Examination of Food Sources of Fibre among High and Low Fibre Consumers. *Nutrients, 10*(9), 1223. doi:10.3390/nu10091223
Belobrajdic, D., Brownlee, I., Hendrie, G., Rebuli, M., Bird, T. (2018). Gut health and weight loss: An overview of the scientific evidence of the benefits of dietary fibre during weight loss. CSIRO, Australia.

52 Fayet-Moore, F., Cassettari, T., Tuck, K., McConnell, A., & Petocz, P. (2018). Dietary Fibre Intake in Australia. Paper I: Associations with Demographic, Socio-Economic, and Anthropometric Factors. *Nutrients*, 10(5), 599. doi:10.3390/nu10050599

53 Eat for Health (n.d.) Nutrient Reference Values for Australia and New Zealand. Dietary Guidelines eatforhealth.gov.au/guidelines/guidelines

54 Eat for Health (n.d.) Nutrient Reference Values for Australia and New Zealand. Dietary Fibre. eatforhealth.gov.au/nutrient-reference-values/nutrients/dietary-fibre

55 Eat for Health (n.d.) Nutrient Reference Values for Australia and New Zealand. Dietary Fibre. eatforhealth.gov.au/nutrient-reference-values/nutrients/dietary-fibre

56 Australian Bureau of Statistics (2014) Australian Health Survey: Nutrition First Results – Foods and Nutrients, 9 May 2014, abs.gov.au/statistics/health/health-conditions-and-risks/australian-health-survey-nutrition-first-results-foods-and-nutrients/latest-release

Fayet-Moore, F., Cassettari, T., Tuck, K., McConnell, A., & Petocz, P. (2018). Dietary Fibre Intake in Australia. Paper I: Associations with Demographic, Socio-Economic, and Anthropometric Factors. *Nutrients*, 10(5), 599. doi:10.3390/nu10050599

Fayet-Moore, F., Cassettari, T., Tuck, K., McConnell, A., & Petocz, P. (2018). Dietary Fibre Intake in Australia. Paper II: Comparative Examination of Food Sources of Fibre among High and Low Fibre Consumers. *Nutrients*, 10(9), 1223. doi:10.3390/nu10091223

57 Eat for Health (n.d.) Nutrient Reference Values for Australia and New Zealand. Dietary Fibre. eatforhealth.gov.au/nutrient-reference-values/nutrients/dietary-fibre

58 Klingert, M., Nikolaidis, P. T., Weiss, K., Thuany, M., Chlíbková, D., & Knechtle, B. (2022). Exercise-Associated Hyponatremia in Marathon Runners. *Journal of clinical medicine*, 11(22), 6775. doi:10.3390/jcm11226775

59 Bajinka, O., Tan, Y., Abdelhalim, K.A. *et al.* Extrinsic factors influencing gut microbes, the immediate consequences and restoring eubiosis. *AMB Express* 10(130). 2020. doi:10.1186/s13568-020-01066-8

60 McDonald, D., Hyde, E., Debelius, J. W., Morton, J. T., Gonzalez, A., Ackermann, G., Aksenov, A. A., Behsaz, B., Brennan, C., Chen, Y., DeRight Goldasich, L., Dorrestein, P. C., Dunn, R. R., Fahimipour, A. K., Gaffney, J., Gilbert, J. A., Gogul, G., Green, J. L., Hugenholtz, P., Humphrey, G., Knight, R., et al. (2018). American Gut: an Open Platform for Citizen Science Microbiome Research. *mSystems*, *3*(3), e00031-18. doi:10.1128/mSystems.00031-18

61 Fleming, A. (n.d.) The British microbiome: how our guts can tell us more than our genes, *BBC Science Focus*, 12 November 2018, sciencefocus.com/the-human-body/the-british-microbiome-how-our-guts-can-tell-us-more-than-our-genes

62 Patangia, D. V., Ryan, C.A., Dempsey, E., Ross, R.P., & Stanton, C. (2022). Impact of antibiotics on the human microbiome and consequences for host health. *MicrobiologyOpen*, *11*(1), e1260, doi.org/10.1002/mbo3.126

63 Virk, M.S., Virk, M.A., He, Y., Tufail, T., Gul, M., Qayum, A., Rehman, A., Rashid, A., Ekumah, J.-N., Han, X., et al. The Anti-Inflammatory and Curative Exponent of Probiotics: A Comprehensive and Authentic Ingredient for the Sustained Functioning of Major Human Organs. Nutrients 2024, 16, 546. doi:10.3390/nu16040546

64 The Nutrition Couch (2023) Leanne's Tips to Beat Bloating, Gas and Constipation. Reviewing ALDI Fit Meals. Susie's Recipe for Wonton Egg Cups. 9 August 2023. https://omny.fm/shows/the-nutrition-couch/leannes-tips-to-beat-bloating-gas-and-constipation

65 Margină D, Ungurianu A, Purdel C, Tsoukalas D, Sarandi E, Thanasoula M, Tekos F, Mesnage R, Kouretas D, Tsatsakis A. Chronic Inflammation in the Context of Everyday Life: Dietary Changes as Mitigating Factors. *Int J Environ Res Public Health*, *17*(11), 4135, 10 June 2020. doi:10.3390/ijerph17114135

66 Farhud DD. Impact of Lifestyle on Health. *Iran J Public Health*. 2015 Nov;44(11):1442-4. PMID: 26744700; PMCID: PMC4703222.

67 Mildenberger, J., Johansson, I., Sergin, I., Kjøbli, E., Damås, J. K., Razani, B., Bjørkøy, G., et al. (2017). N-3 PUFAs induce inflammatory tolerance by formation of KEAP1-containing SQSTM1/p62-bodies and activation of NFE2L2. *Autophagy*, *13*(10), 1664–1678. doi:org/10.1080/15548627.2017.1345411

Bucciantini M, Leri M, Nardiello P, Casamenti F, Stefani M. (2021) Olive Polyphenols: Antioxidant and Anti-Inflammatory Properties. Antioxidants, *10*(7), 1044. doi:10.3390/antiox10071044

68 Visser, M., Bouter, L. M., McQuillan, G. M., Wener, M. H., & Harris, T. B. (1999). Elevated C-reactive protein levels in overweight and obese adults. *JAMA, 282*(22), 2131–2135. doi:10.1001/jama.282.22.2131

69 Cömert, E. D., Mogol, B. A., & Gökmen, V. (2019). Relationship between color and antioxidant capacity of fruits and vegetables. *Current research in food science*, 2, 1–10. doi:10.1016/j.crfs.2019.11.001

70 Ridker P. M. (2005). C-reactive protein, inflammation, and cardiovascular disease: clinical update. *Texas Heart Institute journal, 32*(3), 384–386.

71 Cazzola, R., Della Porta, M., Manoni, M., Iotti, S., Pinotti, L., & Maier, J. A. (2020). Going to the roots of reduced magnesium dietary intake: A tradeoff between climate changes and sources. *Heliyon, 6*(11), e05390. doi:org/10.1016/j.heliyon.2020.e05390

Reynolds, A. N., Akerman, A. P., & Mann, J. (2020). Dietary fibre and whole grains in diabetes management: Systematic review and meta-analyses. *PLoS medicine, 17*(3), e1003053. https://doi.org/10.1371/journal.pmed.1003053

72 Liu, Y. Z., Wang, Y. X., & Jiang, C. L. (2017). Inflammation: The Common Pathway of Stress-Related Diseases. *Frontiers in human neuroscience, 11,* 316. doi:10.3389/fnhum.2017.00316

73 Vlachos, D., Malisova, S., Lindberg, F. A., & Karaniki, G. (2020). Glycemic Index (GI) or Glycemic Load (GL) and Dietary Interventions for Optimizing Postprandial Hyperglycemia in Patients with T2 Diabetes: A Review. *Nutrients,* 12(6), 1561. doi:10.3390/nu12061561

74 Caliri, A. W., Tommasi, S., & Besaratinia, A. (2021). Relationships among smoking, oxidative stress, inflammation, macromolecular damage, and cancer. *Mutation research. Reviews in mutation research, 787,* 108365. doi:10.1016/j.mrrev.2021.108365

75 Khan, N., & Mukhtar, H. (2013). Tea and health: studies in humans. *Current pharmaceutical design,* 19(34), 6141–6147. doi:10.2174/1381612811319340008

76 Kuszewski, J. C., Wong, R. H. X., Wood, L. G., & Howe, P. R. C. (2020). Effects of fish oil and curcumin supplementation on cerebrovascular function in older adults: A randomized

controlled trial. *Nutrition, metabolism, and cardiovascular diseases : NMCD, 30*(4), 625–633. doi:10.1016/j.numecd.2019.12.010

77 Schultz, S., Cameron, A. J., Grigsby-Duffy, L., Robinson, E., Marshall, J., Orellana, L., & Sacks, G. (2021). Availability and placement of healthy and discretionary food in Australian supermarkets by chain and level of socio-economic disadvantage. *Public health nutrition, 24*(2), 203–214. doi.org/10.1017/S1368980020002505

78 Stevenson, R. J., Bartlett, J., Wright, M., Hughes, A., Hill, B. J., Saluja, S., & Francis, H. M. (2023). The development of interoceptive hunger signals. *Developmental psychobiology, 65*(2), e22374. doi.org/10.1002/dev.22374

79 The Nutrition Couch (2021). What Does Your Poo Say About You? All About Emotional Eating. High Protein Wraps and the Low Down on Protein Powders. 10 October 2021. omny.fm/shows/the-nutrition-couch/what-does-your-poo-say-about-you-all-about-emotion

80 Lim Y & Boster J. Obesity and Comorbid Conditions. [Updated 2023 Aug 28]. In: StatPearls [Internet]. Treasure Island (FL): StatPearls Publishing; 2024. ncbi.nlm.nih.gov/books/NBK574535/

81 The Nutrition Couch (2023). Telltale Signs of Fixed Mindsets. Reviewing a New No Added Sugar Chocolate Milk. Susie's Winter Warming Spinach Pie Recipe. 24 May 2023. omny.fm/shows/the-nutrition-couch/telltale-signs-of-fixed-mindsets-reviewing-a-new-n

82 Guglielmo, Beccuti, G., Monagheddu, C., Evangelista, A., Ciccone, G., Broglio, F., Soldati, L., Bo, S. (2017) Timing of food intake: Sounding the alarm about metabolic impairments? A systematic review, *Pharmacological Research*, Volume 125, Part B, 2017:132-141. doi:10.1016/j.phrs.2017.09.005

83 Boege, H., Bhatti, M. & St-Onge, M. (2021). Circadian rhythms and meal timing: impact on energy balance and body weight, *Current Opinion in Biotechnology, 70*, 1–6. doi:10.1016/j.copbio.2020.08.009

84 Lovallo, W. R., Farag, N. H., Vincent, A. S., Thomas, T. L., & Wilson, M. F. (2006). Cortisol responses to mental stress, exercise, and meals following caffeine intake in men and women. *Pharmacology, biochemistry, and behavior, 83*(3), 441–44. doi:10.1016/j.pbb.2006.03.005

85   The Nutrition Couch (2023). Do Meal Times Matter? Why It's Harder to Keep Weight Off After Losing It. The Best Snacks to Have with Your Tea or Coffee. 8 October 2023. omny.fm/shows/the-nutrition-couch/do-meal-times-matter-why-its-harder-to-keep-weight

86   Gudden, J., Arias Vasquez, A., & Bloemendaal, M. (2021). The Effects of Intermittent Fasting on Brain and Cognitive Function. *Nutrients*, 13(9), 3166. doi:10.3390/nu13093166

87   Ming-Li Sun, et al. (2024) Intermittent fasting and health outcomes: an umbrella review of systematic reviews and meta-analyses of randomised controlled trials. *eClinicalMedicine*, 70, 102519, April 2024. doi:10.1016/j.eclinm.2024.102519

88   Kloock, S., Ziegler, C., Dischinger, U (2023). Obesity and its comorbidities, current treatment options and future perspectives: Challenging bariatric surgery?, *Pharmacology & Therapeutics*, 251, 108549. doi:org/10.1016/j.pharmthera.2023.108549

89   Garvey, W.T., Batterham, R.L., Bhatta, M. et al. (2022) Two-year effects of semaglutide in adults with overweight or obesity: the STEP 5 trial. Nature Medicine, 28, 2083–2091. doi:10.1038/s41591-022-02026-4

90   Samuelsson, J., Bertilsson, R., Bülow, E. et al. (2024) Autoimmune comorbidity in type 1 diabetes and its association with metabolic control and mortality risk in young people: a population-based study. *Diabetologia 67*, 679–689. doi:10.1007/s00125-024-06086-8

91   Hall, K. D., & Kahan, S. (2018). Maintenance of Lost Weight and Long-Term Management of Obesity. *The Medical clinics of North America, 102*(1), 183–197. doi:10.1016/j.mcna.2017.08.012

92   Pérez-Gerdel, T., Camargo, M., Alvarado, M., Ramírez, J.D. (2023) Impact of Intermittent Fasting on the Gut Microbiota: A Systematic Review. *Advanced Biology, 7*(8), e2200337. doi:10.1002/adbi.202200337

93   Australian Bureau of Statistics (2023). Alcohol Consumption, 15 December 2023, abs.gov.au/statistics/health/health-conditions-and-risks/alcohol-consumption/latest-release#:~:text=One%20in%20five%20(20.5%25),than%20any%20other%20age%20group

94   Fuhrman, J., Sarter, B., Glaser, D., & Acocella, S. (2010). Changing perceptions of hunger on a high nutrient density diet. *Nutrition journal, 9*, 51. doi:10.1186/1475-2891-9-51

95 Wang X, Ouyang Y, Liu J, Zhu M, Zhao G, Bao W, Hu FB. (2014) Fruit and vegetable consumption and mortality from all causes, cardiovascular disease, and cancer: systematic review and dose-response meta-analysis of prospective cohort studies. *BMJ. 29*(349), g4490. doi: 10.1136/bmj.g4490

96 Manjiang Yao, Susan B. Roberts, Dietary Energy Density and Weight Regulation, *Nutrition Reviews*, 59(8), August 2001, 247–258, doi: 10.1111/j.1753-4887.2001.tb05509.x

97 Foreyt,J. (2012) The Ultimate Volumetrics Diet: Smart, Simple, Science-Based Strategies for Losing Weight and Keeping It Off (Book Review), *The American Journal of Clinical Nutrition*, *96*(3), 681–682. doi: 10.3945/ajcn.112.041418

98 Flood, J & Rolls B. (2007). Soup preloads in a variety of forms reduce meal energy intake. *Appetite*. November 2007;49(3):626–34. doi:10.1016/j.appet.2007.04.002

99 Asif Ali, M., Khan, N., Kaleem, N., Ahmad, W., Alharethi, S.H., Alharbi, B., Alhassan, H.H., Al-Enazi, M.M., Razis, A.F.A., Modu, B., Calina, D., Sharifi-Rad, J. (2023). Anticancer properties of sulforaphane: current insights at the molecular level. *Front Oncol. 13*, 1168321, 16 June 2023. doi:10.3389/fonc.2023.1168321

100 Nottingham Trent University (n.d.) Bacterial fragments from leaky gut help drive obesity, ntu.ac.uk/about-us/news/news-articles/2023/05/bacterial-fragments-from-leaky-gut-help-drive-obesity,-study-shows

101 The Nutrition Couch (2023). Does Your Partner Help Or Hinder Your Health Journey? The Link Between Poor Gut Health and Obesity. How To Enjoy a Morning Coffee While Intermitted Fasting. 13 August 2023. omny.fm/shows/the-nutrition-couch/does-your-partner-help-or-hinder-your-health-journ

102 Shukla AP, Karan A, Hootman KC, Graves M, Steller I, Abel B, Giannita A, Tils J, Hayashi L, O'Connor M, et al. (2023) A Randomized Controlled Pilot Study of the Food Order Behavioral Intervention in Prediabetes. *Nutrients, 15*(20), 4452. doi:10.3390/nu15204452

103 Kubota S, Liu Y, Iizuka K, Kuwata H, Seino Y, Yabe D. (2020). A Review of Recent Findings on Meal Sequence: An Attractive Dietary Approach to Prevention and Management of Type 2 Diabetes. *Nutrients.* 19 August 2020, *12*(9), 2502. doi:10.3390/nu12092502

104 Tricò, D., Filice, E., Trifirò, S., et al. (2016) Manipulating the sequence of food ingestion improves glycemic control in type 2 diabetic patients under free-living conditions. *Nutr & Diabetes*, 6, e226. doi:10.1038/nutd.2016.33

105 Shapira N. (2019). The Metabolic Concept of Meal Sequence vs. Satiety: Glycemic and Oxidative Responses with Reference to Inflammation Risk, Protective Principles and Mediterranean Diet. *Nutrients*, *11*(10), 2373. doi:10.3390/nu11102373

106 Shah, M., Vella, A. (2014) Effects of GLP-1 on appetite and weight. *Rev Endocr Metab Disord* 15, 181–187. doi:10.1007/s11154-014-9289-5

107 Shukla AP, Karan A, Hootman KC, Graves M, Steller I, Abel B, Giannita A, Tils J, Hayashi L, O'Connor M, et al. (2023). A Randomized Controlled Pilot Study of the Food Order Behavioral Intervention in Prediabetes. *Nutrients*, *15*(20), 4452. doi:10.3390/nu15204452

108 Vigil, P., Jaime Meléndez, J.,Petkovic, G., Petkovic, J.P. (2022) The importance of estradiol for body weight regulation in women, *Frontiers*, 13. doi:10.3389/fendo.2022.951186

109 Volpi, E., Nazemi, R., Fujita, S. (2004). Muscle tissue changes with aging. *Current Opinion in Clinical Nutrition & Metabolic Care*. 7(4), 405–10. doi: 10.1097/01.mco.0000134362.76653.b2

110 Pacheco, D., Singh, A. (2023) Lack of Sleep May Increase Calorie Consumption Sleep Foundation, sleepfoundation.org/sleep-deprivation/lack-sleep-may-increase-calorie-consumption#:~:text=Likewise%2C%20lack%20of%20sleep%20can,to%20a%20higher%20calorie%20intake

111 The Nutrition Couch (2023). How to Deal with Weight Loss Plateaus. Reviewing the Latest Healthy Cracker (Olina Seeded Crispbread). Susie's Recipe for Detox Soup. 16 April 2023. omny.fm/shows/the-nutrition-couch/how-to-deal-with-weight-loss-plateaus-reviewing-th

ACKNOWLEDGEMENTS

When we began our podcast, *The Nutrition Couch*, just over 3 years ago, we never imagined we would be here with 5 million downloads to date, and now with our very own book!

There have been many people who have helped us get here. A huge amount of thanks needs to go to our co-founder, David, who patiently edited us for two years and without whom our podcast would not have been possible.

To Bronte Beck, who has been involved in content development from the beginning – so many thanks.

A big thank-you to Tom, who now edits us, and to our brilliant photographer, Dan – you both make us look and sound much better than we do. And to our student dietitians – Tori, Annie and Fiona – thank you for all your help shooting the recipes for this book.

To the team at Penguin Random House, Izzy and Charle, thank you for your vision and for making this process as smooth as possible.

Of course to our families – David, Chris, Gus, Harry, Mia and Matilda – we do what we do for you.

And finally, but most importantly: to our listener family who supports *The Nutrition Couch* every episode. This work is for you. We hope it helps you to reach the goals you have for your health long-term.

INDEX